Realization of the Supreme Self

The Bhagavad Gītā Yoga-s

Trevor Leggett

Postal Address of the Trust:
Trevor Leggett Adhyatma Yoga Trust
PO Box 362
KINGS LYNN
PE31 8WQ
United Kingdom

Website address of the Trust:
www.tlayt.org

First published in 1995 by Kegan Paul International Ltd

Cover designed by Avni Patel

ISBN - 978-1-911467-15-1

Trevor Leggett Adhyatma Yoga Trust

To the late Dr Hari Prasad Shastri, through whom the Gītā speaks for the coming century, this study is reverently dedicated

Contents

PART III ŚAṄKARA ON GĪTĀ PRACTICE

How to use this book for Yoga Practice

You have to know enough theory for a working basis; there is no need to read the subtleties of the intellectual background yet.

THEORY

1. Read Part I, Introductory
2. Read the following sections of Part II
   - (a) Chapter II, Supreme Self
   - (b) Chapter III, Yoga-s of the Self.
   - (c) Chapter IV, Action and *Arjuna's Disbelief*
   - (d) Chapter V, Knowledge
   - (e) Chapter VI, Meditation and *The Thinker, East and West*

MEDITATION PRACTICE

The teaching given in the Bhagavad Gītā is for crisis.

1. Read Part IV, Pointers for Practice

2. Establish a daily rhythm of study, meditation, self-discipline and devotion as explained in the readings. The following is an outline:

Make a firm resolve to do the Yoga practices faithfully for six weeks to give them a fair trial.

Get up one hour earlier to create space for the practices. Set apart a quiet place to do the meditation and study without fail at the same place and time.

Wash hands and feet and sit as described in The Thinker: East and West. Read a holy text for five minutes.

Take several deep breaths and consciously relax the body remaining upright. Make a reverence to Truth. Choose one meditation text from Chapters IX or X for the six week period and focus on it for twenty minutes.

Now practice the Line of Light for fifteen minutes (pages 205 to 211).

For fifteen minutes, visualise an incident from an Avatar's life (pages 199 to 204).

Repeat OM audibly twenty seven times as described by Swami Rama Tirtha (pages 93 – 96).

DAILY LIFE PRACTICE

As practice develops you will find that the contents of Part III will be helpful, especially the Line of Light Section. Once the Line of Light has been established in the meditation period, it can be maintained during the day, at first at quiet moments, and then even in disturbance. It gives many advantages both physical and mental.

Evenness of mind in daily actions is central (page 42 onwards). Independence of circumstances is equally important, appearing in nearly every Gītā chapter (page 193 onwards).

Preface: Experimental Religion

Experimental religion is the method of Self-realization presented in the ancient sacred text called Bhagavad Gītā. Here faith is not blind. Its conclusions, provisional at first, are to be confirmed fractionally in the early experiments; on that basis, faith stretches out to further experiments, in the reasonable expectation that these too can bring confirmations. The method is called yoga, and one who practises it is a Gītā yogin. The practice centres round mind-control in outer life, and meditation within. In time, there is a general inner tranquillization; automatic reactions become fewer and fewer. Free from the tangle of fruitless associations, feelings are integrated, thought and action become clear-cut and effective.

Yoga is a religion in that, at the beginning, God is a hypothesis, not known definitely as either existent or non-existent. He is revered on the authority of others, sometimes reinforced by an obscure inner stirring on rare occasions. After some time, he is dimly perceived as the Universal Lord, a friend and helper of those who worship with faith and purity. After what is usually long practice, he begins to show himself as the essence of man also. First signs are temporary inspiration and then continuous intuition, in daily life as well. It is not necessarily something spectacular. Known or unknown to others, the yogin sees what he is to do in the cosmic purpose, and finds in himself the cosmic joy and energy to do it.

It is easy, and it is not easy. It is easy because the supreme Self is already there. In the depths, beyond local thinking and feeling, beyond the potentialities of local thinking and feeling, there is something calm, immortal and, ultimately, cosmic. That consciousness is called the Supreme Self. It is easy to realize because it is merely a question of getting through unreal obstacles.

It is difficult because these obstacles are felt to be one's very self.

It is easy because a one-pointed devotee is helped by the universal Lord.

It is not easy, because the time comes when that Lord will say to that devotee: 'Give up seeking help from outside. Find Me in your own being, and take your stand there.'

The arrow of the local self has to be shot beyond the gloom of the Unknown into the supreme cosmic Self. The Muṇḍaka Upaniṣad gives the blessing: Glory to you in your flight beyond darkness!

PART I

Introductory

Bhagavad Gītā

Bhagavad-Gītā means literally 'Sung by the Lord'. What are sung are extracts from the Upaniṣad-s, early Indian mystical texts, here put into 700 verses of simple Sanskrit. The Upaniṣad-s had not been taught openly: in the Gītā the secrets are made available to all.

It has been called the Bible of India, but corresponds rather to the Gospels, which contain teachings for everyone's daily life, but also riddling indications of higher truth.

What are these riddles? Surely the message of the Gītā should be simple and straightforward, as is Christ's message of Love in the Gospels? Not so, and not so.

In the Gītā the Lord says: 'Though I have created all this world, know me as one who does no action.' As always in the Gītā, the cosmic declaration has to be applied to the individual also: 'He sees, who sees that all action is performed by Nature alone, while the Self is ever actionless.' Casual readers of the Gītā may not be sure whether this means that some inner self just watches the body and mind being jerked about by Nature like marionettes. If so, it would be contrary to our whole experience, that we do make decisions. Some turn uneasily away from the text. This is why the great commentator on the Gītā, Śaṅkara, says that it can be difficult to understand.

In just the same way some devout Christians mentally turn away from Christ's words on why he systematically taught in parables: 'To those outside everything comes by way of parables, so that (as Scripture says) they may look and look but see nothing, they may hear and hear but understand nothing; otherwise they might turn to God and be forgiven.' The passage comes in three of the Gospels, but there is sometimes a tacit agreement by readers to pass by on the other side.

The Gītā explains why the difficulties are inevitable, and gives practical methods for penetrating to the truth beyond them. In the Indian style, the inspired texts are collated and explained by a commentator, who puts them into precise statements of principle: applications to individual lives are supplied by the living oral tradition. The present book complements the Gītā and its commentary by Śaṅkara with teachings by the late Dr Hari Prasad Shastri from his book *Teachings from the Bhagavad Gītā*. The present author was his pupil for eighteen years.

The Two Traditions

The Bhagavad Gītā (Song of the Lord) is an ancient Indian mystical poem, declaring that the world-process is a divine trick-of-illusion, into which the Lord himself has entered as the inner light of consciousness seemingly held fast in each individual self. He has set himself the problem of struggling free into his universal nature. The Gītā is a revelation from the Lord-in-freedom to the Lords-in-bondage, expounding the truth, and giving the practices for returning to freedom.

The Mystical Tradition

The earliest surviving texts are the Upaniṣad-s, some of them pre-600 BC. They declare the divine origin of the world, its illusory character, the divine manifestation in every element of it, the apparent bondage of the soul, and the methods for attaining freedom. These last are mainly independence of entanglements, search for the divine, leading to profound meditation, then transcendence of the mind in God-realization, culminating in freedom.

The Upaniṣadic sages were experts in practice; they did not fall away into mere theorizing about the Absolute. Ultimately, mental concepts had to be transcended. 'If you think that you know It well' says the teacher to an over-confident disciple, 'little indeed you know.' The disciple goes into profound meditation again.

He returns and says: 'I do not think that I know it well. But it is not that I do not know. He among us who understands when I say that I do not think I know It well, yet it is not that I do not know It, he too knows It.' This is a riddle, and a springboard.

The teachings of the Upaniṣad-s are generally given by Brahmins, the highest class of men whose main duty was to devote themselves to religion, and in some cases to the search for what lies behind religious practice. Still, in even the oldest Upaniṣad-s, the highest teachings are sometimes given by kings to Brahmins who do not know them. That such texts, which show Brahmins as spiritually inferior, were nevertheless faithfully transmitted by them, is a tribute to their integrity. Even when it is a king speaking, however, the situation is one of calm search for truth.

It should be mentioned that traditionally the king was the hardest-working man in the kingdom: his day was divided into eight periods of three hours each. One was for sleep, one for recreation; the rest was for duties – judicial, military, and executive generally. As the Gītā says: 'Of men, the best is the king.'

The profundities of the Upaniṣad-s were put into the verses of the Gītā by an incarnation of the Lord, Kṛṣṇa or Vāsudeva, for the benefit of those still engaged in an active life in society. The formal title of the Gītā is 'The Upaniṣad-s Sung (gītā) by the Lord.' As against the calm atmosphere of the Upaniṣad settings, it is given on a battlefield to a reluctant combatant by another warrior, his non-combatant charioteer. It is not a text of argument, but of revelation and practical instruction.

The Intellectual Tradition

The date of the Gītā cannot be established in the light of surviving historical evidence: some Western analysts believe it is a composite work, because there are contradictions in it. However, the passages adjudged contradictory are often deliberately juxtaposed. They are contradictory only in terms of the pre-suppositions of analysts.

But they are also thought to show that the doctrines are valueless. The point will be looked at later. It is an example of the Fallacy of Fluctuating Rigour: to take contradictions here as proof of falsity, while perforce accepting them for over sixty years at the heart of physics.

There is evidence that in very ancient times, the god Vāsudeva (Kṛṣṇa) and the warrior prince Arjuna were exemplars of a relation of reverence and love – bhakti. In the great Sanskrit grammar of Pāṇini, about 400 BC, there is a sūtra (IV.3.98) to the effect that the suffix -ka indicates devotion in the case of Vāsudeva-and-Arjuna. In theory this might mean that a worshipper of Vāsudeva was a Vāsudeva-ka, and a worshipper of Arjuna was an Arjuna-ka. (Like a Buddh*ist* or a Christ*ian*.) They could each be a separate object of devotion to others. But according to another sutra of Pāṇini (II.2.34), in a compound of two such words, the one with fewer vowels is to be placed first. The word Arjuna has three vowels, while Vāsudeva has four. The fact that Vāsudeva is placed in the leading position, contrary to grammatical usage, shows that the names are not on an equal footing. Vāsudeva is the object of reverence to Arjuna.

It may be mentioned that the early work of grammarians like Pāṇini were masterpieces of analysis, hardly surpassed today. It is a unique phenomenon in cultural history. The Greeks did not make a grammar of their own language till they began to teach foreigners, about AD 100. Nor did it occur to the Chinese to make a grammar; the first was made by the Jesuits, and the same is true of Japanese.

They lacked the passionate interest in analysis of the Indians. (The same was true to some extent of logic. The Chinese translated the main Buddhist texts, and produced many of their own. But they translated comparatively few of the Indian textbooks on logic. They did not believe in exclusive yes-or-no; their outlook was empirical.)

This little grammatical interlude is put in here because it shows the love of precision and subtle corollaries characteristic of the Indian intellectual tradition. The commentators on the ecstatic utterances of the Upaniṣad-s or the Gītā explained every word, and its placing in the sentence, in minute detail. Their ideal was to use words, within their sphere, exactly and logically.

If they had not done this, their works would not have been accepted. They recognized that verbal structures are in a sense self-created and self-creating, and not based on truth. Nevertheless, present life is based on them; it is like an immense edifice of credit. 'The whole business of the world,' says Śaṅkara, 'is based on the prestige of words.' And an ancient Upaniṣadic teacher told the most learned man of his time: 'All the knowledge you have mastered is only a name.'

The Śaṅkara Commentary on the Gītā

Śaṅkara explains the revelatory flashes of the Gītā by putting them side by side with Upaniṣadic texts and with each other. He presents a system which is internally consistent, and which resolves the apparent contradictions of some of the texts. In the end, the system has to be confirmed by practice; it is not a dogma. There has to be enough faith in it to carry out the outer and inner training.

Śaṅkara expects his readers to have a good memory. The traditional method of the commentator was to give an analysis of each word of each verse, and then to show the place of the verse in the whole system. Occasionally he will sum up a particular theme in a long exposition, far beyond the surface meaning of the verse he is commenting on.

Some of the comments, and expositions, are to meet objections by adherents of other schools of thought of his time, for instance Buddhists who held there was no Self, or ritualists. Most of those schools do not exist today, and the arguments and counter-arguments are meaningless for a modern reader. In the Indian tradition of Śaṅkara's time, it was necessary to justify mystical practices by presenting them logically as far as possible. This is much less true of other cultures today. The present book aims to set out the parallels used by teachers, including Śaṅkara, to help and encourage those who wish to train.

The Translation

The Gītā is a book of practical mystical instruction. Though there are descriptions of the world-scheme, it is not an argued metaphysical treatise. The text is in beautiful but simple Sanskrit verse, easy to memorize, and arousing devotion, energy, intuition, and finally peace in the memorizer.

To know exactly what the Gītā text says, read the 1913 Harvard University Press *The Bhagavad Gītā* by Franklin Edgerton, a great scholar who made a special study of this text. He set himself (for the sake of students of Sanskrit) to follow the exact pattern of the original verses, so that each line of the English corresponds to that line of the Sanskrit. In spite of some oddities of English construction, the translation still reads reasonably: in its own terms, it is a masterpiece. Students of the present book are recommended to get the 1972 paperback edition (which omits the Sanskrit). Readers should note that he translated the then little-known word 'yoga' as 'discipline'.

For a modern looser version in attractive English, there is *The Bhagavad Gītā* translated by Juan Mascaro (Penguin Classics).

To learn by heart some key passages of a holy text is one form of the yoga practice of memory. In the present case, Edwin Arnold's old verse translation *The Song Celestial* is not only beautiful but easily memorized.

The present book gives the main points of Gītā practice presented by Śaṅkara, the earliest and greatest commentator. Specific applications to present-day life are mostly from teachings of the late Hari Prasad Shastri, who also exemplified them in his own life. He was a Sanskrit scholar, author of the standard translation of the Rāmāyaṇa epic.

Dr Shastri himself published a small book, *Teachings from the Bhagavad Gītā*, giving some of the important verses with his own comments to them.

The rendering of Gītā verses here is as direct as possible, and in the light of Śaṅkara's understanding of them. Poetic conventions are omitted. For instance, in this type of Sanskrit verse, it was common to use names and epithets to identify speaker and spoken-to: 'O best of men' might correspond to a conventional 'Good Sir' in English. They have mostly been left out, as adding nothing to the instruction. It is however worth knowing that the personal name Kṛṣṇa means Dark, and Arjuna means Bright. What is dark because it is as yet unknown (as Śaṅkara explains), teaches the Bright which thinks all is clear to it.

The reader must expect unpoetic diction, as he would in a training manual. Take verses II.52 and 53 as an example. It reads in Edgerton:

> When the jungle of delusion
>   Thy mentality shall get across,
> Then thou shalt come to aversion

Towards what is to be heard and has been heard (in the Veda).
Averse to traditional lore ('heard' in the Veda)
When shall stand motionless
Thy mentality, immovable in concentration,
Then thou shalt attain discipline.

Edgerton carefully brings out the nuance that this 'hearing' refers to the Vedic texts, many of them ceremonial. But there is an added nuance for the student of yoga practice. These holy texts have been studied with reverence. Some of them are quoted, and others paraphrased, in the Gītā itself. Where does this 'aversion' come from?

The word in verse 52 is 'nirvedam', whose meaning ranges from indifference to loathing. In 53 it is 'vi-pratipanna' which can mean turning from, but also has a sense of being driven to distraction. There is a point when what was taken as good in itself is found to be illusory. If the first commandment endorsed by Christ, namely to love God, is dropped off, the second commandment, to love the neighbour, does not lead to peace. It may be vigorously pursued, but it does not relieve the inner aridity.

Spiritual experience suggests: 'when your mind gets sick of what has been heard ...' and so Dr Shastri sometimes gave it.

In general, the renderings here are not poetical (which often requires context for meaning and effect) but terse and practical. It is the sort of thing found in a training manual, which would prefer 'closed eyes' to 'veilèd lids'. But pupils are urged to read the entire poem, in its original form, to engage the whole personality.

Note on Gender

Following grammatical convention, a singular masculine form means also feminine and plural, e.g. 'The fearless lion was easily wiped out by hunters in Northern India: not so the more cautious tiger.' A feminine form can also be of common gender. A 'sacred cow' includes the bull, which is just as sacred as the cow.

In Roman law, the ordinary Latin word for man, 'homo', could go with adjectives of masculine or feminine form according to the occasion. In this book, 'he' indicates where appropriate: he, she, it or they.

Spelling of Sanskrit Words

There are some Sanskrit words which are not translatable: for instance, samādhi is a meditation state for which we have no English word.

In music, technical terms are internationally understood in the original Italian. As yoga becomes accepted, the few technical terms can best remainin internationally standard Sanskrit spelling. Otherwise Germans will spell Krischna, French Krichna, and the Japanese Kirishina.

It will thus be desirable to adopt the standard system of transliteration. It involves a few extra dots. To learn them is important for a practiser who wishes to use mantra, in which correct pronunciation has an effect on physical energy as well as mental. For the ordinary reader, it means that he can follow easily the wonderful line-by-line literal translation of the Gītā by Edgerton.

Pronunciation

The teacher in the Gītā is Kṛṣṇa. This can sound like Krishna, as in modern Hindi. But the sound of 'ṛ' is more like the 'ur' in 'church'. (In Europe the same vowel is found in Czech: the Czech word for throat is 'krk'. So for millions in the West, this vocalic 'ṛ' sound is easy.)

The dot under the 's' makes it into 'sh'. After getting the 'ṛ', the tongue is already in position for the 'ṣ' and for the 'ṇ'. They are made naturally.

The short 'a', as at the end of Kṛṣṇa, is the commonest sound in Sanskrit. It is not a Continental 'a', but nearer to the short English vowel in 'punch' or 'pun'. Everyone studying Sanskrit is told this, and nearly everyone forgets it. The Victorians were right to spell the common Indian name Hari as Hurry.

After getting to know the few rules, the words will be sounded reasonably well. Once familiar, they can be read from a script without the dots, just as we now read correctly the French word facade printed without the cedilla under the 'c'.

Dots under the 't', 'd' and an occasional 'm', indicate distinctions hardly perceptible to Europeans. The tick above 's' makes it into a light 'sh'. It comes repeatedly here in the name Śaṅkara, which has also a dot above the 'n' of no audible effect.

To sum up:

- ṛ like 'ur' in church
- a like the 'u' in pun
- ā like 'a' in Pa
- ī like 'ee' in knee
- ṣ 'sh' as in gash
- ś light 'sh' as in shilling
- ñ like Spanish señor

- o like Italian 'o': to Anglo-Saxon ears, it has some 'aw' in it; always long as in Ohm
- e 'ay' as in day: always long; Vedānta is not Vedd-anta, but always Vaydahnta

Sanskrit Words and Names

adhyātma	relating to self, individual and finally cosmic
abhyāsa	regular long-sustained practice
Bhīma	'the terrible one'; brother of Arjuna
Bhīṣma	noble general opposing Arjuna's side
Droṇa	noble master archer
guṇa	fundamental element of nature; there are three: sattva (light, truth), rajas (passion-struggle), tamas (darkness, inertia)
jñāna	Knowledge (of highest truth)
jñāna-niṣṭhā	establishment in Knowledge
jñāna-yoga	method of establishment in Knowledge
karma	'action', including its distant effects
Karṇa	heroic half-brother of Arjuna, now opposing him
Kṛṣṇa	partially concealed incarnation of God, who has volunteered to be Arjuna's charioteer
niṣṭhā	taking one's stand on, being established in
Pāṇini	grammarian who standardized Sanskrit about 400 BC
Patañjali	author of the Yoga Sūtra-s

prāṇāyāma	control of vital currents, initially through manipulating breath
samādhi	one-pointed meditation where all associations vanish and the meditation object alone shines out
saṃskāra	dynamic latent impression left by action or intense thought
Sañjaya	sees the battle with divine vision and reports it
vairāgya	serene detachment
Vāsudeva	another name of Kṛṣṇa
yoga	literally 'method'. Spiritual methods to attain Knowledge and then Freedom

The Setting

Queen Kuntī has been given the boon of a night visit in successive years by six gods of her choice. By them she has six sons who are thus half-brothers. Five of them are adopted by her husband King Pāṇḍu, and thus called Pāṇḍavas. The eldest, Yudhiṣṭhira, is to inherit the kingdom. The next two are the fierce Bhīma, and Arjuna who becomes a master archer, and later the disciple in the Gītā. The last two Pāṇḍavas play no part in the Gītā. The other infant, who will be the heroic Karṇa, is abandoned, but found and adopted by a charioteer. This is an important point.

The cousins of the Pāṇḍavas, headed by the cruel Duryodhana, trap Yudhiṣṭhira into a gambling match against a dice sharper; he loses the kingdom to Duryodhana. The Pāṇḍavas are exiled, pursued by the new king's murderous hate. The noble Bhīṣma the commander-in-chief, and Droṇa a great general, who had trained the young Pāṇḍavas, now hold themselves bound by their oath of loyalty to the monarch, though they recognize that the present one is a tyrant.

Another relative of both sides is Kṛṣṇa, a warrior chief who is an incarnation of God, though largely undeclared. He makes attempts to mediate as allies come to support the Pāṇḍavas, but war becomes inevitable. As the armies face each other, Arjuna's will to fight collapses. He suddenly realizes how they will have to kill revered figures like Bhīṣma if they are to win. He appeals to Kṛṣṇa to tell him what to do. Kṛṣṇa makes a few attempts to rally his courage with talk of honour and glory: when Arjuna does not respond, the Gītā teachings begin on an entirely different level.

The teachings begin. But for a long time, as the Gītā will show, Arjuna has his doubts about them. If he had had no doubts, the Gītā would have ended with Chapter III.

The Smile

Arjuna reinforces his refusal, or rather inability, to fight by gilding it with moral sentiments. He presents himself as seeing things from a higher standpoint; from that elevation, he condemns what he had till now wanted to do, but suddenly finds he does not want to do. He had been enthusiastic about the righteousness of the battle, and boasted about what he would do in it. In reliance on his skill and bravery, others had joined his side. Compassion for the members of his family on the other side had not worried him then, any more than it worries his brother Bhīma now. But here he is:

> I.38 Even if they, blinded as they are by greed, do not see
> The sin of conflict within the family
> And the crime of striking at a friend,
>
> 39 Yet we should know enough to draw back from this wickedness,
> When we see what a sin it is to destroy a family.

And further:

> I.46 That I should drop my weapons and be killed on the battlefield, unresisting, by the armed foe,
> Surely that is the better course for me.

Then he makes his appeal:

> II.7 I feel sick at the pity of it, bewildered as to what is right to do;
> I ask you: which is better? Tell me clearly.
> I make myself your pupil; teach me.

How spiritual it seems! But in fact it is not Arjuna's real conviction; it is an excuse for getting out of fulfilling his promises to fight for justice. Kṛṣṇa listens to it not with due solemnity, but with a little smile. He points out the inconsistency of what Arjuna is saying with what he is actually feeling and doing:

> II.11 You are full of pity for people who need no pity at all, and yet you are mouthing words of wisdom.
> Those who have wisdom do not pity either the living or the dead.

Arjuna's words are indeed words of wisdom. They will be echoed in later parts of the Gītā itself. For instance when teaching the high path of knowledge, XIII.7 gives ahiṃsā, harmlessness, as the third of the great qualities to be practised. Nor does Śaṅkara qualify the word when he explains it in his Gītā commentary: 'It means doing no injury to any living being.' This is what Arjuna claims to have realized. But it is not his inner conviction. If it were his inner conviction, he would be wise, and he would not be disturbed by anything that happened.

Those sages who see Brahman everywhere and always are not upset by the changes of the world. They may take part in them, as players take part in a game. In that case, like good sportsmen they try hard, but without being disturbed by the fortunes of the game. On the other hand, sages sometimes set an example to the world by demonstrating absolute pacifism. If they have adopted this role, to them the one who kills and the one who is killed are, so to say, like the right and left hands of the Lord. That, however, is not the role to which Arjuna has committed himself by his actions of the past and his promises for the future. For him now to quote the words of such sages is only self-deception, for he does not in fact feel them. (Kṛṣṇa will point this out again at the end of the Gītā in XVIII.59: 'If from self-will you resolve not to fight, vain is this resolve: your nature will compel you to fight.')

The Lord listens to Arjuna's self-justifications with a half-smile, as grown-ups listen to children talking about things they do not really understand. Boy Scouts may talk about war, and little girls about married life; sometimes what they say is quite sensible, because it is what they have overheard from adults talking. But in fact they know nothing about it.

A clever child who wants to get out of studying grammar can quote some great orator, famous for telling phrases which become bywords in the language: 'When I am speaking, I never think about framing sentences. That would be an obstacle. I simply express what has to be expressed.' Again, a child music student, to escape from practising scales, may cite some famous virtuoso:

'My playing has nothing to do with notes. Notes get in the way. When I play, I have forgotten all about them.'

The novices quote these great ones earnestly. It would be wrong to study grammar: it is an obstacle. It is wrong to practise scales: they get in the way.

The teacher listens to all this with a half-smile, just like the little smile with which the Lord listens to Arjuna's wise words. Then comes the explanation, patient and tolerant: when you are an orator, when you are a virtuoso, when you are a sage – these quoted words will have some meaning. But not till then. In the meantime, you have to learn your grammar, practise your scales, or perform Karma Yoga in devotion and detachment. Admittedly these things are not yet oratory, not yet music, not yet God-realization. But they will lead you there. And then you will realize in yourself the true meaning of what you have been quoting, and you will be able to choose freely what you do.

Kṛṣṇa has the right to tell Arjuna to do his duty and fight. He himself has volunteered to be Arjuna's charioteer, but not a combatant. The charioteer is more exposed than the warrior in the chariot. Kṛṣṇa foresees that he will himself be seriously wounded. Nor has a non-combatant the fury of battle to sustain him, which in the case of active fighters often brings insensitivity to wounds. As for the injunction of ahimsā or harmlessness, on the ordinary level there were exceptions: warriors were to fight in a battle, or to protect the weak, but not for personal reasons. The higher level has to be attained by yoga practice: it is not enough simply to subscribe to it, as Arjuna is finding out. It is given in II.19:

> Who believes him a slayer, and who thinks him slain,
> Both these understand not: he slays not, nor is he slain.

Teaching Down

The usual way of teaching a subject is to build up information to higher and higher levels, each resting on the lower ones, which cannot be dispensed with. It could be called Teaching Up.

But there is another method, *Teaching Down*, for cases where the final knowledge is already there but not recognized. The method is used extensively in the Gītā, and by Śaṅkara following the Gītā. In the Gītā as a whole, first the highest truth of the Self is presented. It is not accepted by Arjuna (as is shown in IV. 4 when he queries the immortality of the Self). Now karma-yoga is given, in very uncompromising form. It has three main elements: (1) enduring patiently the pairs of opposites; (2) performing well directed skilful actions with evenness of mind in success or failure; (3) bringing the mind to complete one-pointedness in samādhi meditation. The whole programme is set out in Chapters II and III. Nothing is said here about devotion to the Lord.

This austere karma-yoga too fails to set Arjuna moving towards freedom from his grief and delusion, and Chapters IV onwards gradually begin to introduce worship of the Lord in various aspects, mostly of an auspicious kind. By Chapter X Arjuna thinks that he has realized truth. But then he asks for, and is granted, the vision of Chapter XI, the Lord as the spirit upholding the Universe, with both auspicious and inauspicious attributes. It proves to be too much for Arjuna as he stands. The Gītā begins again, so to say, with the highest truth and the Knowledge-path. At the end, however, the worship of the Lord is set out to Arjuna again.

The basis of the Teaching Down method is that there is already a submerged intuition of the truth, which has to be stimulated by increasingly detailed instructions. The aim of the instructions is not to give information but to awaken the half-sleeping knowledge.

Plato supplies an example of the method in Western teaching, though what he wants to illustrate is not quite the same.

1. An uneducated slave is presented with a drawing of a square.

2. He is asked to suggest a method of making another square, double the size of this one. His first thought is to double the length of the sides.

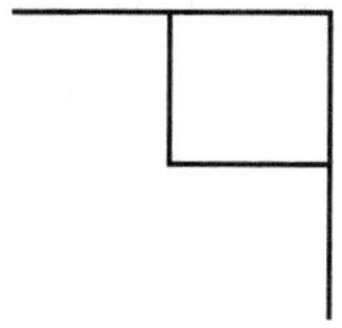

3. This is done, and he is shown how it results in a square four times the original one – consisting in fact of four of them.

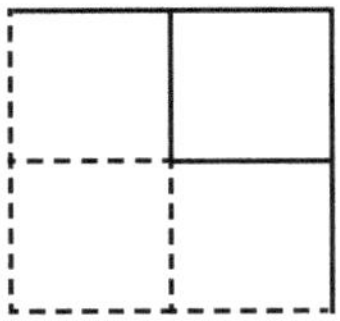

4. It is suggested to him that if each of the squares could be halved, and the halves could make up a square, that new one would be twice the size of the original square.
5. He does not see how to halve a square. A diagonal line is drawn, and he agrees that this halves the square. The shaded area is half the size of the original square.

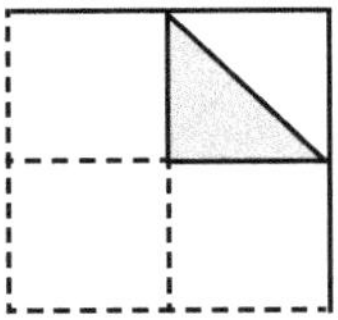

6. Another of the squares is halved with a diagonal line. Perhaps he now says: 'I see it, I see.' If not...

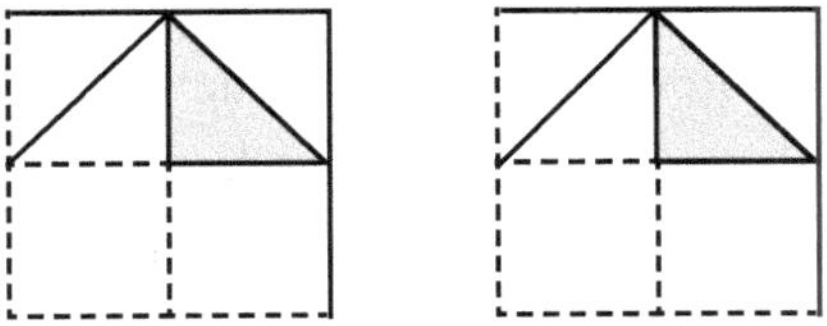

7. Another diagonal line is drawn.

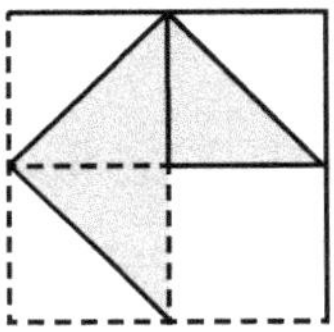

8. If he still does not see, the last one is drawn. If necessary, it is further explained how the shaded square must

be double the original square, because it consists of four halves.

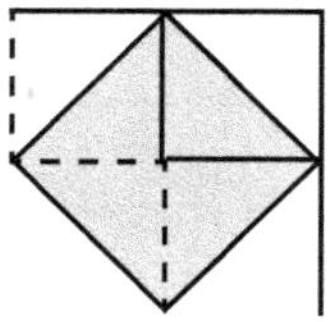

9. At the very end, the extra lines and shadings are rubbed out, and the required square stands out clearly.

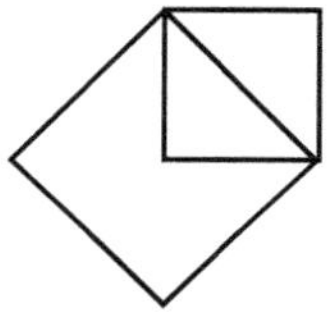

After a time, longer or shorter, he suddenly sees it. Some will have seen it well before this.

It is not a question of learning. The additional lines and shading are not things to be learnt. Nor is it a question of other extra knowledge. Even someone familiar with the theorem that the square on the hypotenuse is equal to the sum of the squares on the other two sides might not see its relevance to the problem of constructing a new square with double the area. The additional lines are to stimulate the intelligence which will ultimately 'see'. The student must not be allowed to think that he is supposed to be learning the new lines; he has to be reminded periodically that the aim is to find a new square.

In a rather similar way, the Gītā first declares the supreme Self, the solution to all grief, hankering and delusion. Arjuna cannot find it in himself; his mind is too disturbed.

So yoga practice is presented to him: calm endurance, acting efficiently but unaffected by results, and samādhi meditation. This is to lead to Knowledge. The process of stabilizing that Knowledge is described – mainly detachment and meditation. This completes the exposition of the path to release (IV.3). Nothing has been said about the Lord as projecting the universe by magic power-of-illusion (Māyā), or about devotion to Him. These are implicit in practice of full realization of the Self, and do not need to be explained separately. It is a fathomless wonder (II.29).

But when Arjuna does not see, Chapters IV and V begin to hint at the Lord as director of the universe, and well-disposed to men, though projecting the divine magic show in which many are deluded.

Karma-yogic action is explained in more detail, but the ideal is also expressed again and again: I do nothing at all – thus should the truth-Knower meditate, though to outward appearances engaged in walking and other actions. Chapter VI gives directions for samādhi, and from VII on there are many declarations of the truths to be meditated upon. In IX and X devotion to the Lord comes in a great flood.

These things can be compared to the extra lines and shadings in Plato's example. They are not always essential, but they do lead to the final realization, in which they can disappear.

Śaṅkara in his commentary frequently makes his explanations in terms of the Gītā teaching method: presenting provisional extra indications where necessary, which later disappear in the full truth.

Part II

Yoga-s of the Gītā

Chapter II Supreme Self

The Gītā is a poem, which sets out the practice for realization of the Supreme Self. That Self is all-pervading, one, unchanging, imperishable, and beyond the grasp of thought. Though it is ever-present, man clings to personal identity, namely restrictions which he thinks are his self. Clinging to limited personality obstructs awareness of the universal Self.

Sometimes it is supposed that a poem, however beautiful, can do little more than create a mood; it cannot give accurate information. This is not so. To take an example from the West: a few years ago, a meteorologist analysed Shelley's poetic masterpiece 'Ode to the West Wind' and concluded that it gave an accurate account of a storm in the Alps, which his own science could not better.

Most of the Gītā consists of instructions given by Kṛṣṇa, who in the fourth chapter – but not at first – declares himself an incarnation of the Creator-Lord. Later, in the eleventh chapter, this becomes an actual revelation seen by two persons, Sañjaya and Arjuna. It is no mere wish-fulfilment, for it has a shattering effect on Arjuna.

Traditionally, the verses are held to be divinely inspired. Details and even contradictions are not poetic licence, but riddles; deeper truths are found by one-pointed meditation on them.

The order of chapters, and the presentation of instruction, is not casual. A special technique is being used, which can be called *Teaching Down*. This kind of teaching is the opposite of building up a body of information and methods of applying it. Teaching Down is concerned with removing illusions. The method is, that the final truth is declared first. If the pupil can 'see' it, and actually embody it, further instruction is needless. If he does not 'see' it, an additional pointer is given, and if necessary further and further indications.

Chapter II, where the teaching begins, is an illustration. The teacher declares the final truth: the one all-pervading, eternal, immutable, fathomless Self. He introduces it with a reference to reincarnation, but makes it clear that it is not a question of a number of individual limited selves being re-born and dying. It is the one Self which is thought to be re-born and die, in many bodies and minds. So how could that eternal changeless One either kill or be killed? Obviously he could not.

> II.12 Never did I not exist, nor you, nor these great men,
> Nor shall we ever cease to be, any of us, in the future.

> 16 What is not, never comes to be; and what is, never ceases to be;
> Those who see the distinction between these two, are seers of the truth.

The doctrine of Illusion (māyā) which plays a big part in later sections of the Gītā, is an expansion of this famous verse (II.16), which is quoted in Śaṅkara's other works also. What does not exist can never come to exist: if it appears, it is an illusion. The illusion may have beauty and meaning, like a picture or stage play, but not if it is taken as absolutely real.

> 17 But know: that is indestructible by which this all is pervaded. That imperishable one, nothing can destroy.

> 24 Neither can He be cut nor burnt, nor wetted nor dried;
> Eternal, present everywhere, fixed, immovable, everlasting is He.

Arjuna hears all this, but he only half believes it, and the Lord goes on in verse 29:

> As a wonder one may see Him, and as a wonder another declare Him,
> And as a wonder another might hear of Him; – but mere hearers do not know Him at all.

An analogy can be a help, though analogies must not be pressed beyond the single point. Imagine a windy day with many moving clouds, and occasional gaps through which the blue sky appears. Small children look at a blue gap and suppose it is a *thing*, which moves, grows larger or smaller, becomes ragged, is cut in two, or destroyed. In fact this is an illusion caused by the movements of the clouds. The sky does not move. Even when the clouds seem to destroy it, in fact they themselves are visible only because of the light of the sky behind them. In the same way the Self appears to be limited by the clouds of the body-mind complexes: it seems to be many, growing larger or smaller, being wounded or killed, disappearing or being born again. In fact these are movements of the mind: the Self is infinite and does not move or change. Meditation on the blue sky is a great yogic means.

Verse 30 completes the indications of the Self. There has been no reaction from Arjuna: in fact he does not believe it, as his question at the beginning of Chapter IV will show. Arjuna feels himself to be a defined personality, and Kṛṣṇa for the moment provisionally accepts this; he speaks of honour and glory, as if rallying the fighting spirit in a temporarily depressed warrior.

But Arjuna does not become fired by the reminders about his honour and ambition: he is becoming more than an ambitious warrior. So Kṛṣṇa goes on to explain briefly something about karma-yoga, the path for those feeling themselves no more than individuals.

Karma-Yoga

The yoga of action, karma-yoga, has three elements: (1) stoical endurance of changes in the world; (2) performance of right actions without laying any claim to their further results (technically called 'fruits'); (3) practice of the profound samādhi meditation, in which mind is focussed and still, undisturbed by anything external or internal.

No efforts in yoga are ever lost, Kṛṣṇa tells him. (This is another piece of instruction which Arjuna does not really accept, as will appear later.)

The first element, brave endurance of the opposites like heat and cold, pleasure and pain, honour and disgrace, is a constant Gītā theme. It is shortly referred to in II.14:

> It is the contacts with material things that cause heat and cold, pleasure and pain.
> They come and go, impermanent as they are; do you endure them bravely.

> II.38 Then treating alike pleasure and pain, gain and loss, Success and defeat, be ready to fight. Thus you incur no sin.

This is the element of karma-yoga called disregarding the opposites. It is just touched on in II.14, where the practice is, to endure them bravely. But in the next verse the Gītā briefly indicates that it is possible to rise completely above them, by realization of the supreme Self. In that case, there is no reaction at all and the yogin is 'fit for immortality'. It does not mean that he does not act: he does move out of the way of a falling tree, for instance. But he does not react, with panic or sighs of relief. Śaṅkara points out that this high state of total independence can be reached even by a warrior in a righteous battle – a battle 'unsought' and therefore defensive, as the Gītā explains.

In the first stage, however, it is not said that the yogin will not feel them; but he must practise keeping his mind even. How is it to be done? One way is to practise focussing the attention on the central line, as described in the Line of Light practice (p. 205). After continued practice, the central line becomes directly felt, and the edge of pain is blunted.

A second aid is to recognize that all these experiences are part of a divine purpose, and accept them as from the Lord. This does not mean not to move away from pain, or not to appreciate well earned rest, but when the pain, for instance, persists in spite of all our efforts, then to accept it as from the Lord, for our own good ultimately. In this teaching, acceptance does not mean to do nothing. The Lord sends the shower; we accept it, and he inspires us to put up an umbrella, as it has been pithily said.

A high form of this practice, for those who are willing to try it, is to look at the experiences, even painful ones, as ultimately imposed by Ātman, one's own self.

As an example: after wartime service, a young man who had hopes of a career in scholarship had a severe stroke, from which he slowly recovered but with the loss of a good deal of eyesight. There was possibility of another stroke. He had practised yoga meditations for some years, and had heard about taking the hardship as imposed by his own Self. He could sometimes attain this, but found it difficult to sustain. Still, it helped him now. Unable to study hard, he managed to find other constructive activity. In addition, every six months he would make an effort at sustained study for a projected book; but after a week, headaches and a sense of risk and doom allowed him to stop without losing too much face to himself. His other activity prospered; he felt he was doing something for the world, and was partly reconciled to his condition. Then an ambitious plan for the future failed – a bitter disappointment. He inwardly addressed the Self: 'How can you put this new disappointment on to me?' In his meditations the reply was: 'You must find my purpose in it.' He felt like shouting at the Ātman: 'You devil! torturing me like this!' He became so angry that he did not care whether he died or not. He pursued the study now through the pain barrier, and in six months completed his first book. It was a considerable success, and laid the foundation for a career. Many years later, he remarked that now, looking back to that time, he felt his younger self shouting at him: 'Why are you torturing me with this new disappointment?' and his older self saying: 'Without it, you would never have taken the risk. I approved of it then and I approve of it now.' The young self says: 'I would have, I would!' The Ātman says: 'No, you wouldn't. And we both know it.' The young one growls: 'You old devil!' and the real Self says calmly and compassionately: 'You young fool.'

If the aspiring yogin has managed, even a little, to make something out of the tragedies and seeming tragedies, he will look back later from the Ātmic standpoint, and say: 'I approve of what happened.' Often what has to be made from it is an inner realization of evenness-of-mind, an ocean in which the little waves which are now so turbulent soon become mere ripples.

> 39 The Sāṅkhya of the Self-knower has been described;
> Now hear about the yoga of the man of action, which can free you from its bonds.

The policy of the Gītā is initiated here: first the direct path of Knowledge (Sāṅkhya) is described, and then – for those who hearing it fail to respond – a more gradual path is given.

> 40 In this course of yoga, there is no waste of effort, nor ever any harmful effect.
> Even a little of the practice saves one from great fear.

> 41 Here, O son of Kuru, thought is one-pointed and decisive:
> Endlessly branching out are the thoughts of the indecisive.

This is the second element of karma-yoga, namely samādhi, where thought is one-pointed and unwavering, identified with the object of the concentration. The one-pointedness is not only the meditation state: when meditation has been practised regularly, the dynamic latent impressions (saṃskāra-s) laid down produce a continuous calm stream of ideas of the truth reached in samādhi. The conclusion reached, or decision taken, does not waver after coming out of that state.

Many-branched are the thoughts of the indecisive. An important factor in training in chess thinking is, not to go over an analysis more than once. Suppose a position where the opponent has moved, and now there are four reasonable replies that might be made. Beginners and medium-strength players look at them in turn, and make a decision: on balance, *this* one looks the best. When about to make the move, suddenly the thought occurs, 'but perhaps that other one might be better if I analysed it again.' Then still another thought comes, and often the thinking becomes quite confused. The final result is an impulsive very bad move, rejected almost at the beginning for a good reason that is now overlooked. Endlessly branching out into doubts and reservations are the thoughts of the indecisive.

The aspiring champion trains himself to look properly at each alternative, and then to stick to his decision firmly. He will not always have found the best move, but at least he will make a reasonable move. And he will not waste his mental energy uselessly.

Still, possibilities are endlessly branching out, so how can one stop the anticipatory thinking also from branching out? How does one know: 'Stop calculating now and stick with the present estimate'? The indication is, that the thinking becomes circular, and pointless. It is true that possibilities are endless, but there is a limit to sensible thinking. When, with no new facts, endless doubts begin to arise, when excuses begin to appear for not going through with a decision already made, that is the time for buddhi to silence the whisperings or ravings of instinctive mind (manas) and emotional mind (citta). When the regimen prescribed by the doctor becomes irksome, manas will say: 'After all, he may not be right. The treatments prescribed by doctors 100 years ago now look silly, even harmful; in 100 years' time, this treatment of today may look equally silly, even harmful. Perhaps I should trust my own inner feeling.' Buddhi says: 'No! we have taken the decision on the best advice available, and we stick to it. Silly inner feelings are what got us into this bad state of health in the first place, and we don't trust them now. In this yoga thought is one-pointed and decisive.'

It may be added here that the whole idea of self-control and tranquillizing the mind is opposed by some theories of today (some of them based on deliberate misreading of Freud). It is said that feelings should be respected, and expressed, not slighted and repressed. There is a fantasy that if everyone acts freely on impulse, it will be Paradise. In fact, the strong, the beautiful and the cunning would finally get everything, leaving others destitute. The Gītā shows that there is no lasting happiness without control of impulse, feeling and thought. Acting on impulse sometimes gives instant satisfaction, but it also lasts only an instant and is followed by a reaction in the form of depression. Many of the talented and persuasive Joyous Vitalists, like Jack Kerouac, and Jack London in former days, died early of alcohol poisoning.

Feelings too are of various kinds: they must be controlled. If inordinate attachment is not controlled, fear and anxiety will not be controllable either. In the Permissive Society, anxiety and depression are endemic, as is shown by the doctors' prescriptions, and widespread use of harmful drugs (including alcohol).

There follow three verses (42–44) on the after-death states promised by the Veda-s for those who perform the sacrifices. These ceremonies included feeding the poor, and donations to learning, and had some social meaning. But they were for the restricted personal benefit of the sacrifices and as such are dismissed by the Gītā. The states of heaven and hell are as real as the present world – that is to say, based on illusion but with some coherence. The experiences in them are the results of actions here, good and bad. Hell can be compared to agonies of hospital treatment to someone who has shattered his body by drug abuse or fighting; a heaven has been humorously compared to being permanently drunk in a night club on an apparently unlimited expense account. All these states are passing, and ultimately sources of suffering because they are restrictions.

> 47 Your right must be to the action alone, never to its fruits,
> Let not the fruit of action be your motive, nor be attached to inaction.

> 48 Set in yoga perform your actions, casting off attachment;
> Be the same in success or failure; this being-the-same is called yoga.

Being the same in success or failure does not mean slackness in action. Throughout the Gītā, the word in these passages is 'kārya', which means 'what ought to be done'. It is sometimes translated 'duty', but there is some difference. In kārya the sense is that the action is done for its own sake, not under compulsion, nor to get some personal advantage. It is done with enthusiasm and zest, as actualizing the cosmic purpose in one small area, but not for personal gain. The karma-yogic skill in action is not indifference to the action: it is indifference to fruits.

Śaṅkara makes this a central verse of the Gītā. Arjuna does not have an option, he cannot chose between the paths of Knowledge and of Action, namely between jñāna-yoga and karma-yoga. He is simply not qualified for the path of Knowledge; he would not be able to follow it, inasmuch as he is still subject to grief and illusion. His qualification is for action alone. The word for qualification is adhikāra, which means something like a proper role, a qualification, with the added sense that it ought to be done as fitting, as a proper duty.

Then three important points are given about the actual performance of yogic action as distinct from ordinary action of the world:

1. No claim on the fruits of the action. For instance, no feeling of injustice if it is successfully done, but someone else reaps the benefit.
2. The motive for action is not to be connected with fruits. This is not the same as (1). To do an act of charity to get self-satisfaction would not be yogic action. A test would be, that the act is immediately forgotten by the giver.
3. 'Not be attached to inaction,' This very important half-line is to rule out a common mistake. The mistake is: to confuse acting yogically without being attached to the fruits, with making sure there is no attachment to fruits by doing nothing, so that there are no fruits. Nearly everyone at some time makes the slip of glossing over careless action, or inaction, by thinking: 'After all, I am a yogin, I am not working for results.'

The yogin *does* work for results. But they are not the reason why he undertakes the action, nor does he have any claim on them. He does the action because it ought to be done, whether it succeeds or not; he is not elated if it comes off, nor cast down if it does not. But he always acts as efficiently as possible to bring about the best result. Later in Chapter III, the Gītā will say that the ideal action is 'yukta', namely well-directed, and Śaṅkara glosses this word as meaning efficient and well chosen.

All this is summed up in verse 50, which also links up with the next verses on sitting-in-meditation samādhi:

> He whose mind is thus held in yoga of evenness,
> Casts off here the vice or virtue of actions;
> Therefore devote yourself to yoga:
> Yoga is an art of skilful actions.

In II.48 yoga was defined as evenness of mind, and here it is further described in regard to actions, as a skill and an art. How is that evenness to be attained, so that it will inspire skilful action? The next verses describe yoga in itself, namely samādhi meditation. It may be noted that the word 'yoga' and associated words such as 'yukta' come many times in the Gītā text, and in most cases Śaṅkara glosses them by 'samādhi' or associated words such as 'samāhita'.

> 52 As your mind gets through the tangle of delusion,
> You will get sick of all you have heard and what you are still supposed to listen to.

> 53 When your mind, bewildered by the traditional lore,

At last comes to stand motionless, immovable in samādhi,
You will have attained yoga.

This is a passage with wide meaning. To study the holy texts is a sacred duty, like giving in charity and virtue generally. But if it is done without meditation, it leads to a kind of frustration. Reading the lives of the saints, for instance, without practising meditation oneself, is humorously compared to counting the money in someone else's pocket. In the same way, virtue practised without inspiration leads to contradictions. Feed the starving, heal the sick: does this include feeding and healing mass murderers? What about their future victims, when they are fit and strong again? Mother Teresa of Calcutta remarked that social service done without prolonged periods of prayer in silence is good work, 'but it is not Christ's work'.

The translation should if possible reflect the situation: something has been done with enthusiasm, but is finally found to be pointless by itself, as Śaṅkara says. 'Get sick of' is a harsh colloquial phrase, but it is meant to mirror a harsh direct experience of disillusion. It was used by Dr Shastri of this situation.

The two verses on samādhi apply to both karma-yoga and knowledge-yoga, but there is a distinction as regards what it is centred on. The calm concentration of the karma-yogin is directed to some element in his yoga, such as independence, or evenness of mind; or the One Thought of verse 41. This last will be some aspect of what Dr Shastri used to describe as the established Master Sentiment – often some aspect of God. All these are facts-within-the-world: there is an independence deep in the heart, there is an evenness also. Then supporting and controlling the world are the great manifestations of the divine. They cannot be seen clearly until samādhi is attained. But after it has been practised for some time, they begin to show themselves, though not perfectly clearly, even through the veil of the world-experience, when it is thin. When it thickens, the yogin practises samādhi again. The same applies to the knowledge-yoga. Until consciousness of time and place are transcended, Brahman, the Ātman-Self, is not seen. But when it has been seen in samādhi, it can be seen outside samādhi, when body and mind are active. There is a description of the state in IV.24, when the actions of the remaining body-mind have taken on the character of an offering into the sacred fire of Brahman, the universal Self:

> The act of offering is Brahman, Brahman is the offering itself;
> it is put into the fire of Brahman by Brahman;
> He whose samādhi realizes action to be Brahman, will go to Brahman.

In verse 54 Arjuna asks about the steadying of Knowledge. He knows from experience of life that even clear Knowledge can be clouded or disturbed by past associations, though they are known to be unreal. How is it to be recognized that the Knowledge has been stabilized? He asks for a description of what a man of steady Knowledge is like externally. How does he speak, how does he sit, how does he move? (He clearly has some doubts about Kṛṣṇa as a model. The point will be looked at later, under the section called Arjuna's Disbelief.) Disregarding the slight, Kṛṣṇa answers:

> II.55 When he gives up all desires in the mind,
> And is satisfied by himself in the Self alone,

He is said to be one whose Knowledge has been steadied.

56 When his mind is not disturbed by sorrow,
And he has lost the desire for joys,
Without hankerings, fears or anger,
The sage is said to be firm in Knowledge.

57 When he has no desire for anything,
And when something good or bad comes to him,
Neither delights in it nor repels it,
His Knowledge has been steadied.

58 And when he withdraws his senses from objects,
As a tortoise withdraws all its limbs into itself,
His Knowledge is steadied.

Why does the Knowledge have to be steadied? In his commentary on II.17 and elsewhere, Śaṅkara explains that the idea 'I am not the body-mind; I am the true Self' is still an idea. It is founded on truth, but the expression in words or thoughts is an affair of the mind. The mind is now pure and clear, so that truth can be reflected in it. But it is not truth itself. The thought 'I am Ātman' is not Ātman. Ātman has no need to think: it knows everything already, because it is everything and also transcends everything. The thought in samādhi ('I am Self') destroys illusion of identity with limited body-mind. So it destroys itself also, since the very thought is part of the mind. Ātman, the universal Self, alone remains.

But the Knowledge-idea has to be steady before it dissolves in Ātman. It can be disturbed by a sudden rush of sense-impressions and memory-associations.

> 60 The impetuous senses can carry off the mind of even a Knower,
> Though he is struggling to control them.
>
> 61 Then let him sit and make samādhi on the Self, and so restrain them.
> As his senses come under control, his Knowledge is steadied.

The Gītā says repeatedly (for instance in V.23, or here in II.70) that such impacts from the senses continue as long as life lasts, but they can be controlled. The karma-yogin controls them by meditating that they are illusory, and sources of suffering in the end; he also practises overruling them by rousing his Master Sentiment. The Knowledge-yogin does it by samādhi on the Self.

Much more serious is the case where people allow themselves to meditate on the sense-objects themselves, even though they may restrain the actions of desire. It may be very difficult to disentangle the mind from cherished fantasies. Still, as the Gītā promises, it can always be done by one sufficiently disillusioned, and determined to change.

In the final state of steady Knowledge, such sense impacts make almost no impression at all:

> 70 Just as the sea remains ever undisturbed, though the rivers are endlessly pouring into it,
> So is the sage at peace from desires,
> But not the one who lusts after them.

71 He who moves about without desires or longings,
With no self-interest and no feeling of limited 'I'
He goes to peace.

72 This is the state of Brahman;
Once attained, delusion is no more.
If one finds this even with his last breath,
He goes to Brahman.

This chapter summarizes the highest teachings. No God apart is described; Self is one. Even the karma-yogin is expected to find strength in himself: within him, as within all, is the one Self, the Lord infinite in power and infinite in daring, as Chapter XI will describe him. Śaṅkara however softens the presentation by bringing in some of the elements of devotion to a Lord felt as separate, which will come in later chapters.

Chapter III Yoga-s of the Self

The third chapter has more on the two paths, and particularly action, including self-interested righteous action which is not yogic at all. Near the beginning there is a description of the principles of performing largely ritual sacrifices as worship of the gods, in the justified expectation that they will make a return in the form of blessings and prosperity. This is the assumption that underlies the Book of Job, but is transcended in the final vision. The Gītā refers in a number of places to such beliefs, sometimes with guarded approval. (The present day recognition of ecology, and even the Gaia hypothesis, are belated acknowledgement of the importance of reverence for nature.) But it points out that they are not yoga. They lead only to improvement of outer circumstances and sometimes of inner ones also. They do not free from the prison of individual separateness, with its consequent desire, fear and grief.

Chapter III expands the account of karma-yogic action. Four types of bond have to be let go: anticipated results as a motive for action; attachment to results, anticipated or actual, as a personal claim ('Why has God let us down?'); attachment simply to being active; attachment to inaction (often masked as leaving everything to the Lord's will).

> III.4 Not by not initiating actions does a man attain freedom-from- action;
> Not by renunciation alone, does he go to perfection.
>
> 5 For no one can remain totally without doing actions even for a moment;
> Everyone is forced by the guṇa-s of Nature to engage in action, whether he wishes it or not.
>
> 19 Therefore do what needs to be done, remaining unattached,
> For acting without attachment, one attains the highest.
>
> 20 For through action alone, Janaka and others attained perfection.
> Moreover, for the support of the people, you should do action.

Usually the Gītā does not analytically separate out the first three, though in certain cases the distinction is made. In any case, action of karma-yoga is done because it ought to be done, and it is done in evenness of mind irrespective of the results seen.

The karma-yogin performs the action from his individual self, vigorously taking his part in the world but trying to give up his personal reactions.

The word 'kārya' – what-is-to-be-done – shows that the action is done for its own sake, not for personal gain or from fear or pressure.

These are verses praising right action as both inevitable and also beneficial. Yet in the middle of them, comes a verse which seems to contradict the whole thesis:

> 17 But the one who takes delight in the Self alone, who finds contentment in the Self,
> And satisfaction in the Self alone -
> For him there is no action that needs to be done.

It is a feature of the Gītā presentation that the two standpoints, one of not-Knowing and the other of Knowledge, are put alongside each other. The reason is that one of them – karma-yoga – is in the end based on illusion. Were they strictly separated off, aspirants might well tend to attachment to karma, without wanting even to hear about anything else.

The other type of action is no-action; it is the seeming action of the true Self-Knower. In this case it is realized that Self does not act; body and mind act, but now the actions are free from distortions caused by limited individuality. It has to be conscious awareness, not a mere idea of non-action which is contradicted by present experience at every step. The purified body-mind complex acts under divine direction to help others, materially also, but mainly towards Self-realization for themselves.

> 25 The fools act who are attached to action;
> And like them should the Knower too act, but without attachment,
> For the good of the people.

The Knower is cautioned not to upset those attached to action as absolutely real. His surviving body-mind complex sets an example of unselfish detached action. But he does not bewilder them by talking about rising above action. But we should notice that the Knower's actions are done with the same intensity as those of one seeking results at all costs. They are not slackly performed. But inwardly there is no attachment; as a sort of spin-off, the actions are more efficient. They are not distorted by the personal considerations which constrain ordinary actions. The actions are done in conformity with the nature of the instruments, and not of the agent. Hence they are done with love, and not unnaturally forced.

As often in the Gītā, the chapter ends with a warning. Here is repeated the warning of II.60, that even Self-knowledge and realization can be clouded by desire and anger. They must be overcome by repeated samādhi, said Chapter II, by which in the end mind itself is transcended and the Self is realized beyond the mind. But the recommended practice seemed circular: samādhi was to cast off desire and anger, but desire and anger would prevent samādhi.

This chapter explains that the casting off can be gradual. The mind has to be recognized as higher than the senses: long-term aims are achieved only by checking immediate impulses.

Then the buddhi or rational will is higher than mind: long-term desires are evaluated, and it is realized that purely selfish satisfactions involved pain for oneself and others. With increasing inner clarity, there are flashes of Self-cognition, and desires begin to be seen as tawdry and unreal in comparison. But desire finally ends on full Self-realization: 'only when he sees the Supreme does his longing finally cease.'

There is almost nothing in this chapter about devotion to the Lord, or about the glories of divine manifestation, which play such a big part in many later chapters. Here the stress is still on the highest truth of Self, universal and quite apart from body-mind. The theme of the bliss of the Self is brought forward: verse 17 speaks of delight in the Self alone, and satisfaction and contentment in the Self alone. The Sanskrit word 'rati', delight, is very strong; it is not a mere cessation of suffering, but positive bliss independent of any object. There is a nuance of sportfulness about the word.

The highest realization of Self does not impede completion of action already entered on before the rise of Knowledge. But such action is free from personal ties, and so is usually highly efficient. Here is a description of karma-yogic action:

> 30 Consigning all actions to Me the Self, with full self-awareness,
> Free from longing and from selfishness, fight, casting off your fever.

The actions are offered, so to say, to the Self, as an act of faith, for the Self is not yet directly known. 'Self-awareness' in this verse still refers to the individual self. The word is 'adhyātma', and Arjuna later on, in Chapter VIII, asks what exactly it means, and is told it is his own nature as he stands. (Śaṅkara points out that this limited self is ultimately going to be realized as the universal Self.) Individually initiated actions of karma-yoga are recognized as having value: they thin out the mind-tangle. But ultimately it is a question of Self-realization, beyond even the most refined layers of the mind.

With this, the yoga has been fully expounded, says Kṛṣṇa (IV.3).

Arjuna's Disbelief

In typical traditional pictures of the Gītā scene, Arjuna is shown with palms joined in reverence, looking at Kṛṣṇa in an attitude of devotion and faith. But this is not what is described by the Gītā itself, in which Arjuna shows from the very beginning that he does not really recognize Kṛṣṇa as a teacher or as a god. For a long time he has little confidence in what he is told. There is a series of indications, which can, however, easily be overlooked.

It is a great advantage to readers today that the doubts are brought out so clearly. There is a tendency to think: 'Oh, in those times they had absolute faith in what they were told: of course that's not true for us today.' In ancient times there was just as much scepticism as today. Already in the time of the Buddha (fifth century BC) there were influential schools, with thousands of followers, who taught that religion was a confidence trick of priests. Some said further that there is no such thing as virtue or sin: 'if a man slaughters hundreds of innocents, burns and pillages, he commits no sin: if he saves hundreds of lives and is compassionate to all, he attains no merit. Borrow money, and do as you like.'

Though Arjuna was a religious man, he was quite capable of thinking for himself, and so the Gītā text makes clear. The teaching begins in Chapter II, in response to an appeal by Arjuna:

> II.6 We do not know which is worse for us, that we should conquer them, or they should conquer us;
> If we killed these noble men who stand arrayed against us, we ourselves would not want to go on living.
>
> 7 My very soul is tortured by weakness of compassion, and I am bewildered as to what I ought to do;
> Now tell me definitely which is the better course. I make myself your pupil: teach me.

This last is usually taken as establishing a guru-disciple relationship. (The traditional requirements of an offering, and doing some service, are assumed to be waived in a crisis, as indeed the texts allow.) But Arjuna himself demonstrates, almost immediately, that this is far from the case. Having just now said: 'Tell me what to do,' he adds (verse 9): 'I will not fight.' As so often when spiritual advice has been sought, there is an unspoken assumption that it will, indeed must, confirm a decision already made. Arjuna's physical condition shows that it is not a question of deciding at all; he *cannot* fight. His limbs collapse, his whole body shakes, he drops the bow; his skin burns, he cannot stand still, his eyes are blurred with tears. So in reality he wants approval for his decision based on his present condition.

In fact Kṛṣṇa does not at first give spiritual advice at all, but points out the disgrace of Arjuna's not fighting after having boasted of what he will do. 'Think of what they will say: how they will laugh! The great warrior running away!' This is to test, for Arjuna himself, whether it is merely a momentary depression, such as all fighters feel at times, which can be dispelled by appealing to their ambition and honour. If Arjuna returns to fight on this basis, he will be like all the others: a loyal warrior, but not a yogin. Only when these worldly considerations (which are repeated two or three times) have no effect, does Kṛṣṇa begin the instruction on yoga, by declaring the final highest truth, the transcendental Self:

> II.17 Know that that is indestructible by which all this is pervaded;
> Nothing can destroy this imperishable One.

Arjujna hears this, but does not really believe it, as is shown by his question in IV.4, when Kṛṣṇa has just said that he declared this yoga at the beginning of creation. 'That was long ago,' objects Arjuna, 'and you are here now: how can I make sense of this?' In other words, he does not believe it. Kṛṣṇa has called him a 'devotee', but that devotion is still with reservations.

Sometimes they surface much later. In II.40 Kṛṣṇa has presented karma-yoga, with the encouraging words:

> In this there is no loss of a start once made, nor does any reverse occur;
> Even a little of this practice saves from great danger.

But in VI.37 Arjuna puts forward his doubt:

> An unsuccessful striver whose mind, though endowed with faith, falls away from the practice without completing it – what happens to him?

Experienced teachers know the situation well: when a pupil for some reason does not want even to try, he says: What will happen if I fail?

> Fallen from both, does he not perish like a wind-torn cloud,
> Without any basis, gone astray on the path to Brahman?

Arjuna has not believed what was said: 'In this there is no loss of a start once made, nor does any reverse occur.' So Kṛṣṇa has to explain at length how the dynamic power of yogic efforts once made will finally carry their performer onward, even though he may temporarily resist.

Arjuna can express his incredulity quite bluntly. A little earlier in this same Chapter VI, Kṛṣṇa has shown him how to meditate, but the pupil objects:

> VI.34 I do not see how the meditation as you have described it can hold steady for long;
> Mind is changeable, impulsive, powerful and obstinate;
> To try to hold it would be like grasping the wind.

Kṛṣṇa indicates briefly what he will develop later: by laying down dynamic latent impressions through regular practice, and lessening the force of distractions by seeing clearly what they are, mind can be controlled.

Arjuna then moves at once to his second line of defence, mentioned above: 'What happens if I fail?'

Sometimes Arjuna's disbelief is shown by his total lack of reaction. For instance, in Chapter X the Lord is giving special manifestations in which he is to be seen most easily, and he refers to the tribe of the Vṛṣṇis of which his present body as Vāsudeva is a member, and also to the group of five Pāṇḍava brothers, of which Arjuna is one. He declares:

> X.37 Of the Vṛṣṇis I am Vāsudeva, of the Pāṇḍavas I am Dhanañjaya, and of the saints I am Vyāsa, of the sages I am Uśanas.

Arjuna's nickname, as a master archer, was Dhanañjaya, 'winner of gold prizes'. Here the Lord is saying: 'I am you.' It is like one of the Great Sayings of the Upaniṣad-s: 'You are That.' But Arjuna shows no reaction at all. It simply passes over him, like some poetical fancy. This is what Śaṅkara refers to when commenting on X.20, where the Lord declares that he is the Self in the heart of every being. Śaṅkara points out that some cannot yet meditate on the Self. So for them the Lord gives external glories, such as 'I am Vyāsa of the sages', 'Himālaya of mountains', 'OM in the Veda-s'.

There are the reverse cases where Arjuna *thinks* that he believes absolutely, but has unconscious reservations still to be brought out.

He says at the beginning of Chapter XI that having heard these statements of glory, he believes them absolutely and his delusion is gone. He does not know that the greatest ones – 'I am the Self in the heart of all beings' and 'Of the Pāṇḍavas I am you' – have completely escaped him. In the last third of the Gītā, Chapters XIII to XVIII, they will be presented in various ways so that they can be gradually accepted, and the limitations of individual self dissolved in the greatness of its true Self.

There are many other hints in the Gītā that Arjuna regards Kṛṣṇa as less than perfect. At the end of Chapter II he asks him about the one whose Knowledge is firm: 'How does he speak, how does he sit, how does he walk?' Similarly at the end of Chapter XIV he asks: 'What are the marks of one who has transcended the guṇa-s? How does he behave?' These are extraordinary questions to ask when he has a perfect example right in front of him of the perfections he is asking about. The Gītā mentions them to show that some passing shadowy hesitations and doubts can continue for a long time. It also shows that they are all finally dissolved into space.

How Arjuna Addresses Kṛṣṇa in the Gītā

In XI.41 Arjuna begs forgiveness for (among other things) having used familiar language in addressing the Lord: 'Kṛṣṇa' 'Yādava' (descendent of the Yadu tribe, equivalent to 'Scotty', etc.) This, and the change after seeing the Universal Form, are illustrated by the terms in the Gītā itself.

I.21	Acyuta = firm one (also not leaking away, not falling, etc)
28	Kṛṣṇa (lit. black)
31	Keśava (lit. hairy)
32	Govinda – cow-herd
	Kṛṣṇa
35	Kṛṣṇa – slayer of demon Madhu
36	Janārdana – jana (men) ardana (distributer); excitant, stimulator, nuisance, gadfly

37	Mādhava: related to spring, vernal; descendant of Madhu
39	Janārdana
41	Kṛṣṇa
	Vārṣṇiya – Vṛṣṇi clansman
II.4	Madhu-sūdana
54	Keśava
III.1	Janārdana
36	Vārṣṇiya
V.1	Kṛṣṇa
VI.33	Madhu-sūdana
34	Kṛṣṇa
37	Kṛṣṇa
39	Kṛṣṇa
VIII.1	'Best of men', Puruṣottama (no Śaṅkara comment: not supreme Spirit here)
X.12	Supreme Brahman, supreme Light, supreme Purifier; eternal divine Puruṣa, primal God, unborn Omnipresent
X.14	Keśava
	Lord (bhagavān)
15	Puruṣottama (here supreme Spirit), source of beings, Lord of beings, God of gods, ruler of the world
16	all-pervading
17	Yogin
	Lord
18	Janārdana
XI.2	Lotus-eyed (kamalapattrākṣa)
3	Supreme Lord (parameśvara), supreme Spirit

15	Description of Universal Form
24	O Viṣṇu
25	O Lord of Gods, abode of universe
30	O Viṣṇu
36	O Lord Supreme
36	Hṛṣikeśa (lord of the senses)
37	Mighty Being, primal Cause, infinite Being, Lord of gods, abode of universe, imperishable, Being-not-being, supreme Lord of gods
38	Primal God, ancient Puruṣa, supreme abode of all, knower and knowable and supreme abode, all-pervading, of infinite forms
40	Infinite in power, infinite in daring
42	Acyuta
43	Greatest Father of the world, etc.
	guru (only time this word used in Gītā for spiritual teacher, though Bhīṣma and Droṇa are gurus of strategy, archery, etc.)
	Here in XI.43 it refers to the Universal Form which terrifies Arjuna and which he asks to be removed.
45	God of gods, abode of universe
46	Thousand-armed, Universal Form
XIV.21	Prabhu (lord)
XVII.1	Kṛṣṇa (!)
XVIII.1	Great-armed
	Hṛṣikeśa
	Slayer of demon Keśin
73	Acyuta

Chapter IV Action

The chapter begins with a statement by Kṛṣṇa that the ancient yoga has now been taught. Elaborating on a single word – purā, of old – in III.3, he gives briefly its history. He taught it to the first king, and it was handed down through king-sages (not through priests, an important point). This account Arjuna immediately pronounces impossible. The first king-sages were in the distant past, but Kṛṣṇa is here now, so he could not have taught it to them. How can I make sense of this? he demands.

Kṛṣṇa replies that he has had many births, and so has Arjuna also. I know them all; you do not know, because (adds Śaṅkara) your natural omniscience is obstructed by your binding acts of right and wrong. This interchange shows that the Gītā does not teach narrow worship of Kṛṣṇa, that being merely one birth out of many. Nor is it a cult of Viṣṇu worship, in which it is Viṣṇu who enters the divine incarnates. There are only three references to Viṣṇu. One is as a minor deity, in X.21; and in Chapter XI the terrifying aspect of the Lord is twice addressed as Viṣṇu. The God of the Gītā is universal and transcendental, the true Self beyond all names. It is not far from the I AM of Exodus 3.14.

Following the principle of Teaching Down to a dull or sceptical pupil, the Lord now speaks of something different: his own true unmanifest being, from which the universe has been projected by magical illusion (māyā). He says that he enters into it periodically as an avatāra or descent, to adjust it physically, morally and spiritually.

Arjuna makes no comment, and Kṛṣṇa goes on to present the supreme action of world-creation and maintenance as a model for human action. It is done without yearning for some hoped-for fruit. This is as far as most humans will be able to go. But there is a higher level still, the level of Knowledge: it is done without a sense of 'I do it'. Following the Teaching Down principle, the supreme level is presented first, and then the provisional lower level. Verse 13 running on into verse 14 goes:

> Although I am the doer of all this,
> Know Me as one that eternally does no act.
>
> Actions do not taint Me, for I have no yearning for any fruit from them;
> He who realizes this of Me, is not bound by actions.

The man of Knowledge should be like this: a doer, but no doer. Such phrases can become mere clichés as Śaṅkara points out, and the actual practice will be examined later.

The second verse gives Kṛṣṇa as a model for men who have not yet attained Knowledge, who feel themselves acting: they can free themselves by abandoning desires for the fruits of action. This 'abandonment of fruits' can also become a cliché, if not fully penetrated into.

Again, phrases like 'although I am the doer, I am one that does no act' may sound like nonsense, or a mere poetic fancy. An illustration from daily life can be useful. In the ordinary way, no one thinks 'I breathe'. When I have been sitting still, I say that I was doing nothing. A sleeping man does nothing, though in fact he still breathes. But flung into water, non-swimmers just try to get the head out of the water, they don't think 'I breathe'; they simply want air. Poor swimmers too are always trying to climb out of the water. They too do not think 'I breathe'. One who is training to be a swimmer is made to lie face downward in the water to realize that the body floats: then he practises the strokes, turning the head regularly to the side in order to breathe. Such trainees are very conscious of breathing, and results do not seem very good; they take in water and have to stop, spluttering. As they become expert, everything becomes easier: the forward movement produces a hydrofoil effect, and finally the breathing becomes regular and drops out of conscious awareness. They no more think 'I breathe' than does a man on land.

The yogic parallel is that the free Self does not act. But having in sport thrown a ray of itself into the sea of not-Knowing, there is individuality which seeks only self-preservation. It does not think 'I act'; it just wants gratification of its desires. When it begins to train, it acts consciously, following a discipline which often does not seem very attractive. But with practice, a sort of spiritual hydrofoil effect makes actions easier, and finally they drop away from conscious awareness. (This is only an illustration, and cannot be pressed too far.)

A new element that has been introduced, for Teaching Down, is the Lord as a model, both for men of Knowledge-realization and for those who have not yet got it. It is a gesture of the Gītā that action is recommended for the Realized as well as for the others who are still acting on a basis of 'I am the agent'. In the case of the Realized, the recommendation is addressed to the suffering body-mind alone.

> IV.23 Rid of attachment; freed, his mind fixed in knowledge,
> Acting simply as a holy offering, his whole action melts away.
>
> 24 The act of offering is Brahman, Brahman is the offering itself; it is put into the fire of Brahman by Brahman;
> He whose samādhi realizes action to be Brahman, will go to Brahman.

In the last part of the chapter, the Lord explains in detail various practices of worship and also control of the life currents, by which men of action purify themselves for Realization. The true culmination is always to be Knowledge-realization, whose practice in samādhi is the highest purification.

Verse 34 is the only passage in the Gītā on seeking a teacher. The teacher must be one who knows not only theoretically but also by direct experience. He must be 'established in Brahman' (brahma-niṣṭhā).

> Learn to know this from those who have knowledge and see the truth:
> Revere them, question them, serve them; and they will teach you knowledge.

This passage is treated in full in the chapter called 'The Spiritual Teacher', p. 291. The chapter ends with a warning especially against doubt. It is to be cut by Knowledge, as are other impurities. Even the worst of sinners is completely purified by Knowledge-realization. (The same will be said later of devotion to the Lord.)

> 36 Even if you are the worst of sinners,
> You will cross the ocean of sin by the boat of Knowledge.

> 38 For there is no purifier to be found here that is equal to Knowledge;
> He who perfects himself by yoga, finds it in time in himself.

Chapter V Knowledge

Readers are advised that Śaṅkara in this chapter uses technical terms and concepts to establish his position on knowledge. On a first reading it does not have to be studied in detail.

The Lord has said in IV.3 that the highest secret of yoga has now been taught. Nevertheless he has to continue to explain it in different ways because Arjuna has not fully accepted it. As is said at the very end, the Gītā will continue till Arjuna can understand, and incorporate it into his own being.

At the beginning of the chapter Arjuna asks one of his questions, which show he has no clear idea of what he has been told. This time it is about the Two Paths. Kṛṣṇa answers that for one who has not yet seen the truth, the path of action is better, meaning (says Śaṅkara) that it is more feasible for him than the knowledge path of those who have glimpsed the Self. Even if a man of action attempted the path of knowledge, he would still feel that he was a limited body-mind self, and that to go beyond action, he must literally give up his home and live by begging. This would be no more than outer imitation of someone like the Buddha. Inside, he would be boiling with frustrated impulses and ambitions. (In historical fact most of the ancient preachers, even of the crudest materialism, were expected to practise this sort of outer austerity in order to get a following.) In the Gītā view, this kind of life may properly be practised by some, but only after knowledge has been attained. Otherwise, though renouncing outwardly, he will still be attached inwardly, for instance to reputation as a great renunciate.

As a rough summary of the many passages, there can be three main renunciations:

1. Physically giving up action, or at any rate all actions except begging as a sort of reflex. This may have nothing to do with the internal feeling; such a man might be full of suppressed impulses to action. The car has been stopped, so to say, but the engine is still running.
2. Karma-yoga renunciation:

   of personal motives,

   of attachment to results ('fruits') of action, of busy attachment to action itself,

   of attachment to inaction. (This last may be disguised as submission to the will of God.)

   In the renunciation of karma-yoga, the yogin is still firmly held by the sense of 'I do', and convinced of the absolute reality of the world.
3. Knowledge-yoga renunciation:

   This is transcendence of the living feeling: 'I am a doer, busy in a world of many real things.' Stepping out of this feeling is the renunciation of the truth-knower. Body and mind continue in illumined action, under the light of knowledge, but there is no feeling of 'I do'.

Most of Chapter V, especially from verse 17 to the end, describes the yoga of Knowledge, says Śaṅkara. The path is not a question of trying to reinforce knowledge. Once that has sprung up, it needs no effort of reinforcement. The phrases used are 'steady knowledge', 'firm knowledge', 'unwavering knowledge' and the like. The path, pursued with effort, consists in giving up trailing memory-associations which may obscure knowledge. In form it is a positive injunction. In Śaṅkara's words: 'Knowledge Yoga (jñāna-niṣṭhā) is an intent effort to maintain the current of knowledge'. But really it is negative. An example would be an instruction to a gardener: 'Keep the stream running.' That does not mean somehow pushing the water along by paddling the hands; it means, not letting dead leaves or rubbish clutter it up. The stream will run naturally if not interfered with. This is a central point in Śaṅkara's Gītā presentation.

Śaṅkara calls the path of Knowledge jñāna-niṣṭhā, literally 'taking one's stand on Knowledge'. It is no mere theoretical idea, for Śaṅkara repeatedly calls it also samyag-darśana-niṣṭhā, taking one's stand on Right Vision. Or again he gives it as paramārtha-darśana-niṣṭhā, taking one's stand on Vision of the Supreme. This knower is a Seer and his direct Vision qualifies him for the knowledge-path called jñāna-niṣṭha. (The translation 'devotion to knowledge' may fail to make it clear that it is already attained.)

The process of jñāna-yoga is mostly meditation on the supreme Self as free from all trails of obscuring cloud, which may arise from memories and past associations. Though known to be illusory, they can still have an effect. The same thing happens in life. Someone who has lived under a tyranny but is now in a very free country, can feel an irrational fear when talking to an official.

The official may be seen and known to be helpful; but there is a deep-seated suspicion, arising from memories. It is known to be unreal, but yet creates an internal spasm. Special treatment may be needed to get over the unfounded fear. Similarly the yogic realization may need time to dispel unreal convictions of limited identity. The yogic current finally comes to continue in all mental states: active, withdrawn, or sleeping.

Verses 8 and 9 are a typical Knowledge text. The meditation is a natural continuation of Knowledge in the body-mind complex, which survives till death. The natural train of knowledge need only be left alone, and not interfered with. Interference could come from pondering on memories of deceptive promises of sense-contacts, as II.67 has warned. The text here shows that it is mainly a question of not falling back into the illusion of being a scheming doer and a keenly personal experiencer.

> V.8 'I do nothing at all' – thus should the truth-knowing yogin meditate, even when seeing, hearing, touching, smelling, eating, walking, sleeping, breathing,
>
> 9 Talking, throwing out, grasping, opening and shutting his eyes – ever affirming: 'All that is merely the senses acting on sense-objects'.

It must be noticed that this is directed to a 'truth-knower', who has a sight of the Self. His Right Vision will continue of itself so long as he does not become distracted from it. As one Teacher put it: 'He who has once got out of a place should not turn and smile smugly at what he has left. If he does, he may find himself back in it again'.

The Gītā extends the general statement to all activities, even to fighting in the case of a warrior-king such as Kṛṣṇa himself. It echoes the verses in Chapter II (which themselves echo the Kaṭha Upaniṣad):

> II.21 He who knows as indestructible and eternal this unborn immortal one, how could he slay, and whom could he cause to slay?

The truth-knower's body and mind act directly under the divine impulse, which also controls the results according to the divine purpose. The mind of a Knower is to meditate all the time: 'I do nothing at all', as verse 8 says.

Verses 8 and 9 teach Knowledge-yoga. Then unexpectedly and abruptly verses 10–12 bring in a karma-yogin. This man is 'performing action' (though without attachment), whereas the truth-knower was meditating 'I do nothing'. Before the direct experience of Self, a yogin still feels 'I am doing this'. In his case, he has to throw away attachment to the fruits when he acts, but is not yet able to throw away the sense of 'I do'. He is referred to in the verses:

> V.10 He who acts without attachment, casting his actions upon Brahman, evil does not touch him, any more than water a lotus- leaf.

> 11 With body, mind and intellect, and even with the mere senses, the yogins perform actions, giving up attachment, in order to purify themselves.

> 12 The yogin, abandoning the fruits of action, comes to abiding peace; the one without yoga, acting from desire, is attached to the results, and so is bound.

But the very next verse speaks of him when he has truth-realization of the Self:

> 13 Mentally abandoning all actions, he sits happily, as the lord in the nine-gated citadel of the body, neither acting nor causing to act.

It seems deliberately confusing that the two standpoints, so completely opposed, are put side by side, so to speak. It is typical of the Gītā teaching method that the two stands (niṣṭhā) come in consecutive verses. One has sympathy with Arjuna's complaint: 'You are confusing me'. Why doesn't the Gītā put the karma-yoga passages neatly together in one section, and the Knowledge-yoga in a separate one? Then it could say: 'When you have at last mastered this karma-yoga, you will be ready for Knowledge-yoga' – that would be logical and clear.

Or so it seems. But in fact it is based on a wrong notion. If this were done – and it is sometimes done unconsciously by disciples – many people would consign themselves to karma-yoga for good. Who could boast of having mastered karma-yoga? The At Last would become Never.

The Gītā teaching method seeks to prevent this. It is true that the two standpoints are opposed, but the point is, that this opposition is an illusion. It is strong, 'hard to get over' as the Lord says. But it is not a solid fact. A long-held illusion normally takes a good time to dispel; but it can also drop away in an instant, just because it is only an illusion. It has no solid basis.

Still, an illusion may be persistent. Most people have to make a number of tries before they can comfortably handle a snake, even though they know this one is not venomous. There are however a few, equally repelled at first, who suddenly manage to drop their aversion. With most of us, it fades away only gradually. The Gītā states twice that the change may be quick, though not necessarily correspondingly easy. Some Teachers believe it is a question of courage.

Under verse 12 Śaṅkara sets out the programme of the two paths:

1. karma-yoga samādhi, on renouncing action by not seeking its fruit, then
2. purity of essence, leading to
3. attainment of Knowledge (jñāna), then
4. renunciation of actions, and
5. steadying Knowledge (jñāna-niṣṭhā), and lastly
6. mokṣa, freedom.

He repeats this programme often, sometimes shortening it by, for instance, putting Knowledge-renunciation and Knowledge-steadying together. He emphasizes (under verse 26) that it is the Lord's programme, repeated by the Lord in the Gītā 'at every step', constantly.

The chapter is mainly on Knowledge, and it gives some of the effects, (or lack of effects) of Knowledge:

> V.18 In a learned and pious Brahmin, a cow, an elephant, a dog, a vagabond, the sage sees the same.

This does not mean that he would not bow to the Brahmin, or would not give something to a starving beggar. He will follow his role, as an actor does in a stage play. Outwardly he conforms to the distinctions, but inwardly he sees them all as members of the company.

The chapter develops the brief phrase in II.55: 'content in the Self by the Self alone':

> 21 When his self is not attached to outer contacts, and he finds happiness in the Self; when he is set firm in Yoga, he attains imperishable bliss.

> 24 He who finds his happiness within, his joy within, and so also his light within, that yogin becomes Brahman, and goes to Brahman-nirvāṇa.

The nouns in these passages are strong: sukha is the ordinary word for happiness, and words like rati (joy) are from the root ram which has a sense of positive delight, with a nuance of sport, like the English 'disporting oneself'. It is more than mere cessation of suffering.

> V.25 Brahma-nirvāṇa is attained by seers whose sins have been destroyed, doubts cut away, senses controlled, and who delight in the welfare of all beings.

Brahma-nirvāṇa is explained by Śaṅkara as freedom absolute, and the seers of the verse are men of Right Vision (samyag-darśin).

Verse 25 speaks of delighting in the welfare of all beings, a phrase that comes twice in the Gītā text. It is echoed in XVIII.45

on karma-yoga, where it speaks of delighting in the dharmic exercise of innate qualities. In Knowledge-yoga, it will refer to that same action, but under divine impulses, without the feeling of 'I do'.

The next few verses of the chapter sum up knowledge-yoga, which follows the purification effected by karma-yoga. Jñāna-yoga is in fact the last three steps of the whole path. Śaṅkara sets them out here, as he did under V.12. They are (1) Attainment of Knowledge (jñāna-prāpti), (2) Steadying Right Vision (samyag-darśana-niṣṭhā), (3) Renunciation of actions (saṃnyāsa). We see that jñāna-niṣṭhā of V.12 is here given as samyag-darśana-niṣṭhā, showing that the Knowledge is not theoretical, but direct experience of Right Vision. For those qualified for it, knowledge-yoga is the short course, the direct path to freedom absolute.

There is a warning (22 and 23) about anger and desire. As long as life lasts, traces of these may appear in the mind of even a Knower. The Gītā repeats this several times, for instance in III.39–41. It happens even though they are known to be unreal, just as even adults can become exultant or angry over the effects of a trivial game. They know it is all unreal but still they are excited by the apparent gain or loss. This is not to say that a spiritual adult never has anything to do with things of the world, but he must know what he is doing. The Gītā warns that he must not seek his pleasure in them. As many verses say, he must be able to withdraw the senses and fix attention on Self as Brahman in samādhi meditation.

Śaṅkara stresses that knowledge in a form such as 'Here I am, free' is not yet freedom. It is a mental operation, and complete freedom entails freedom from all mental operations, as explained at length in Chapter II. Knowledge, he says, leads to freedom by way of destroying illusion. While there is knowledge as an idea, freedom is not complete. We find a hint in the examples given above. Suppose someone living under a tyranny escapes, after many dangers. For several days, such people think all the time: 'Free, free', and cannot in fact do much else. They are free, and they have also the idea of freedom. The idea itself in a way hampers their freedom. When it is fully incorporated, they do not think 'I am free, free'. They simply are free, and exercise their freedom in any way they like, active or at rest.

Chapter V ends by outlining the technique of sitting meditation, to be given in further detail in Chapter VI. It has two forms: (1) realization of freedom, and (2) meditation on God for purification. (1) is described first:

> V.27 Shutting out the touch of the world, and with gaze fixed between the eyebrows, making the in- and out-breaths pass through the nostrils evenly,
>
> 28 Controlling senses, and lower and higher mind, the sage, with freedom as his goal, without desire, fear or anger
> - who is ever thus, is free.

The Thinker, East and West

It has been an axiom for thousands of years in the Eastern traditions that the body reflects the mind, as the mind reflects levels deeper than itself.

Rodin's 'Thinker' is here side by side with the 8th Century clay figure of a Chinese Lohan or Buddhist saint. Both of them have been thinking, but what a great difference! In fact, the wonderful technique of Rodin conceals the unnaturalness of the posture. Most people, asked to sit like the famous 'Thinker', put their right elbow on the right knee. They are quite surprised to find out that it should be on the other knee, an uncomfortable position that cannot be held for more than a short time. The knuckles of the right hand are pressed so hard against the mouth that the lips are pushed out of shape. In spite of the apparent calm of the pose, the figure is expressing inner agony, appropriate perhaps for one looking at the gate of hell. (That is the original setting.)

Rodin's Thinker conveys his acute observation that most people do not know how to think. In this bronze it is as if the thinking faculty were calling on the physical body somehow to help, by distorting itself. The mind cannot simply think; it demands that the body should play a part too. But it cannot tell the body what that part should be, and the body does not know what it is expected to do. So it twists and turns in frustration. Rodin's genius conveys this too: very soon, the Thinker will have to move. The body twist will slip, and the pressure on the mouth will become too uncomfortable. There are other points in the posture showing its inherent instability. And apart from the physical discomfort, he will want to move anyway, to relieve momentarily his inner disquiet.

The Eastern thinker by contrast is well balanced and at ease, in body and nerves. The limbs are drawn in and centred, and the head is balanced on the spine. There are further advantages obtained from a traditional posture like this one, but they are best learned from experience.

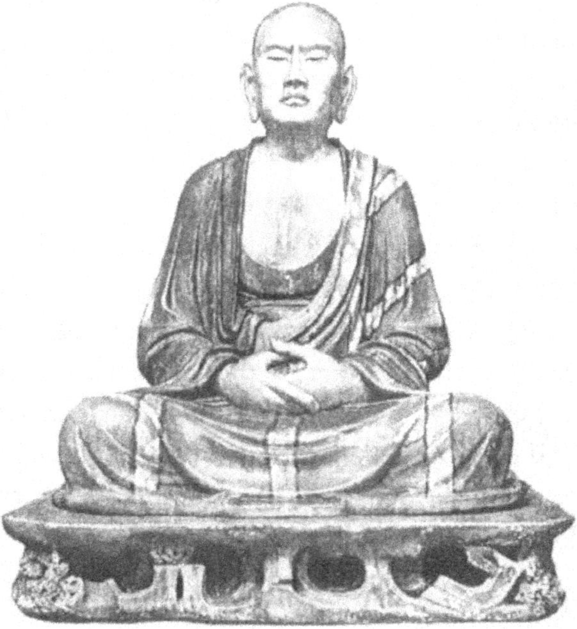

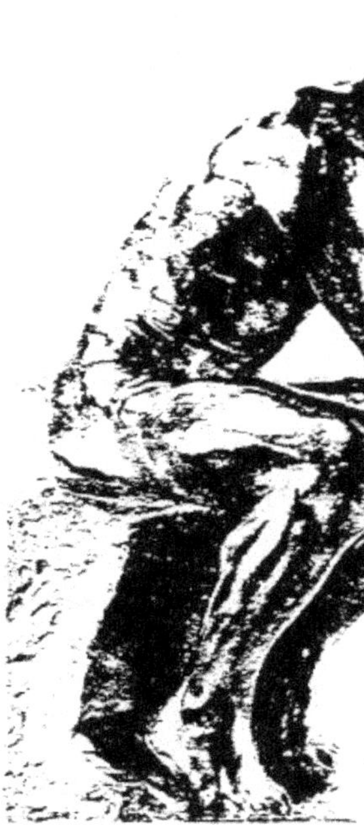

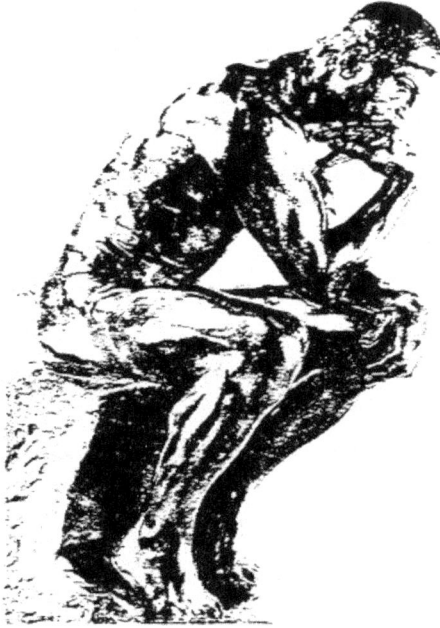

It takes most Westerners (and a good many Easterners too) some time to acquire a good posture. In actual practice, the half-lotus is generally used. This can be attained by a normal person under thirty in six weeks. If the muscles have shortened from habitual chair-sitting, this position can be conveniently acquired outside the meditation period. Sit morning and evening for thirty minutes on a folded blanket on the ground. Draw in the legs, and put one foot on the opposite thigh, the other being tucked under the hips. Read a spiritual book, and the moment there is any pain, take down the foot, and put up the other one instead. Alternate the feet in this way for the thirty minutes, having a short rest period if necessary.

Slowly the knee of the uppermost leg will ease itself down, till it rests on the ground. Young people notice the discomfort at first, then cease to notice it, and finally after three months find the position so comfortable that they may fall asleep in it.

As soon as the position is tolerable for half an hour, it should be adopted for meditation proper.

Before taking the formal sitting position, it is a good idea to stretch the limbs. This does not imply the contortions of the so-called hatha-yoga, which is a late development, probably about the seventeenth century AD. One of its main purposes (as can be seen from some of the inducements to practice mentioned in its basic texts) is to improve the functioning of the physical and prāṇic instruments, and it often leads to intensified identification with them. The traditional yogic practices are to secure reasonably good health so that the body does not disturb meditation and ordinary life. There are formal stretching exercises, which were taken from India to China, but these too can become a mania. For most people it is sufficient to imitate the stretchings of a cat when it wakes up. The limbs are extended and then flexed, in turn, and then the whole body, and head and neck.

For the meditation proper, a reverence is made, and then the seat taken. The hands are usually lightly clasped, the abdomen pushed a little forward, and the chin drawn in without strain. It is important to take exactly the same posture each time. The body becomes used to it, and settles more comfortably into it. After training for some time, the adoption of the posture has itself a calming effect on nerves and thinking process.

On the same principle, it is best to sit in the same place, and at the same time every day. There are many advantages in establishing a regular rhythm, in meditation as in other things. When an athlete practises every day at the same time, about half an hour beforehand his blood pressure begins to go up, and the muscle tone improves, in anticipation of the exercise. On days when his body is fatigued, the current of practice carries it along without much effort. Similarly a regular meditator will begin to experience an inner pacification even before the formal sitting begins.

While life happens to be flowing fairly smoothly, one may feel that one has no need of such devices. As so often in spiritual training, the thought comes: I should be free, free, free. Nevertheless, it is worth adopting them, making use of the experiences of the experts of the tradition. Many of us find that when circumstances become really turbulent, we are not quite so tough as we thought we were.

There are schools which lay great stress on formal posture. Many yoga schools however recommend simply approximating to it, and then doing one of the Line of Light practices. This produces what is technically called an up-stroke, which spontaneously pulls the body up into a good posture. As this comes about of itself, to fuss over it is only a distraction. And in fact meditation on God does itself bring about good posture along with other advantages: 'From devotion to the Lord comes perfection in samādhi', says Patañjali's Yoga Sūtra.

One of the purposes of the meditation posture is to lead to transcendence of the body-consciousness (Yoga Sūtra 11.45). To be slumped in an armchair is not in fact relaxation: there is constant shifting, and inner tension even when not moving. Good meditation posture is a sort of knack, which gives a sense of opening and expansion: poets have compared it to an infinite blue sky.

Chapter VI Meditation

Chapter VI is on meditation technique. It speaks both to the karma-yogin, the man of action for whom samādhi is only one of the three parts of his training, and then to the Knowledge-yogin, for whom it is the main part. In fact, for the Knower it is natural that mind remains in samādhi while life lasts; the only effort for that mind (but it can be a considerable one) is to keep away from following mirages of past associations.

The whole tenor of the chapter is self-effort: 'let one raise himself by himself, let him not degrade himself' (verse 5). But there is a difference in the means for the two stages:

> VI.3 For him who is still trying to attain yoga, acting is said to be the means; for the same, when he has attained yoga, quietening is said to be the means.

Before he has reached samādhi on the Self, while he is a man of action involved in the world, yogic action, without personal motives and making no claim as to the fruits, is what he has to do. It makes his mind transparent, and he will finally attain

Knowledge of Self, as it springs up in his direct experience. After that, the final means to liberation is to stay at peace in the serenity of Self-realization, till the last traces of restriction to a limited personality die away.

The karma-yogin is to practise in daily life the actions proper to his role, in an unselfish way. To do this he will have to free himself gradually from bondage to external things and inner compulsions. Instructions are given on meditation which will help him to do this. The karma-yogin's meditation is not on the Self (he cannot do that yet) but on some holy object:

> VI.10 Let the yogin practise yoga in a secluded place,
> Alone, restraining thought and mind; free from hopes and any feeling of possession.
>
> 11 Let him in a clean place lay out a steady seat for himself, not too high and not too low;
> Let him put on it a grass mat, and over that a skin, and over that a cloth.
>
> 12 There let him fix his mind on a single object, and rein in the activity of mind and senses;
> Sitting on that seat, let him thus practise yoga for self-purification.

Purification means thinning the tangle of the inner apparatus of mind and causal body; as they become transparent, there are glimpses of the Self beyond, seen at first as an awesome wonder.

Hints are given for keeping the meditation steady:

> VI.13 Let him sit firmly, keeping straight and still his body, head and neck, not looking at anything else but the nose-tip.

Westerners (and some Easterners) often do not care for the nosetip gaze. It is however found in most of the schools of meditation, not only in India but in China and Japan also. A very restless mind can be pacified by controlling the pupils of the eyes, and this is one of the methods. However, it usually needs instruction and encouragement from a teacher to carry it through. A modern teacher, Dr Hari Prasad Shastri, recommended it to some pupils.

> 18 When his controlled thought rests on the Self alone,
> Free from hankering after any desire,
> That one is called a yogin.
>
> 19 It is said of the yogin whose mind is controlled in the yoga of Self, that it is like a flame burning calmly in a windless place.
>
> 20 When thought comes to rest, checked by yoga practice,
> When, contemplating Self by self, he is at ease in the Self,
>
> 21 When he knows that supernal joy which is beyond the senses but appreciated by the higher mind,
> And never deviates from it but abides steady in it,
>
> 22 Which having gained, he realizes it as higher than any other gain,

And having been established in it, he is not shaken even by great pain,

VI.23 This yoga-yoke, let him know, is an unyoking from misery.
It has to be practised with determination, and without being daunted by difficulties.

Little by little this is practised, and not by sudden violence. If force is used there may be a temporary exaltation, but usually followed by an equally violent reaction. Violence in this technical sense includes drugs, unnatural postural distortions, screaming excitement, very rapid breathing, self-torture and compulsory asceticism, and so on.

26 When something tries to distract the fickle and unstable thought process, it must be drawn back by the higher mind and fixed again on the Self. Then let him go beyond thinking.

This last sentence is the inhibition (nirodha) of all mental operations. Often teachers do not insist on it much at the beginning because it seems like suicide to those who identify thought with consciousness. In the yoga experiments, thought is found to be only a movement in consciousness. But until there is some experience, it is imagined that consciousness without thought would have to be just a blank.

The nirodha state beyond thought had been described much earlier than the Gītā in the ancient Bṛhadāraṇyaka Upaniṣad, and much later in Patañjali's Yoga Sūtra-s. In fact many of the technical terms of Patañjali's yoga are found already in the Gītā. Śaṅkara's commentary on it is full of them.

The results of yoga practice are given: the infinite joy, already mentioned in Chapter V, appears again and again, and now there are indications that it is the great Self that is appearing as the Lord:

> 29 The yogin settled in samādhi sees the Self in all, and all in Self;
> He sees the same in everything.
>
> 30 For that one who sees Me in all, and sees all in Me,
> I am never lost, and he is not lost for Me.

Having heard the instruction on meditation, Arjuna breaks in with the objection that it is impossible – like trying to grasp the wind. The teacher explains that it is indeed difficult, but can be done by regular practice, and detachment. The words used – abhyāsa and vairāgya – are quoted in Yoga Sūtra 1.12: 'Their inhibition is by practice and detachment.'

Arjuna then displays a momentary will-to-fail (familiar to teachers of anything at all) by asking what happens to one who drops out of the training. Does he not lose both worlds, this and the next? Kṛṣṇa patiently expands the phrase in II.40: 'There is no loss of effort here.' Such a man will be reborn in favourable circumstances for yoga practice, and the dynamic latent impressions of his former practice will forcibly bear him onwards, 'whether he wills it or not'.

An indication is given at the end about meditation on the Self as the Lord, and this is to be developed in the beautiful verses of Chapters VII, IX and X.

Chapter VII The Lord

Chapters V and VI have been mainly on samādhi-meditation. For karma-yogins, it was described as performed by individual effort: for Knowledge-yogins, it is a natural continuation of their realization. The four chapters that follow, VII to X, are mainly for karma-yogins who cannot find the resources in themselves to control their passion or inertia. They are to regulate the feelings by concentrating them on the Lord, whose perfection will naturally attract and refine them.

At the beginning of Chapter VII, the Lord states that the revelations now given are to be understood theoretically, and then experienced practically in yoga meditation. What is first a matter of faith must become direct experience.

An example is this. The Lord describes his projection of the world, and says that he is its dissolution too. He continues:

> VII.7 There is nothing higher than I;
> On Me all this is strung, like chains of pearls on a string.

The simile is one of faith, but not of blind faith. One of the points is, that the string is invisible, being hidden by the pearls strung on it. But a second point is that the string is known to be there; otherwise the pearls would not remain in order but would be scattered. In the same way the order in the world shows that there is an underlying intelligence which holds it together, which integrates it. Perhaps some scientists are beginning to recognize this. And if the pearl chain is minutely examined, there are tiny glimpses of the string. There are such glimpses of the cosmic string in meditation, and perhaps in some delicate experiments in physics which have puzzling results.

The Lord goes on to describe himself as the essential quality in things – the taste in water, light in moon and sun.

> VII.9 Both the fragrance in earth and the brilliance in fire am I;
> Life in all beings, and austerity in ascetics am I.

Śaṅkara interprets this chain of verses in another, deeper sense, as describing what the yogin sees when his meditation has been successful. He says that it becomes a unity: it is not that austerity in the ascetics is visible (like the pearls), and the Lord inspiring it is invisible (like the string), but that the Lord is both the austerity and the ascetics practising it: 'In Me as austerity the ascetics are woven.' In this realization, the 'pearls' are really knots in the string itself, which from a little distance look like separate things, held together by something underlying them.

In III.27–29 there was a brief mention of the three strands or energy-qualities (guṇa) of material nature (prakṛti). The Lord now describes in detail, with beautiful similes and illustrations, this nature. It is divine, and he calls it his māyā (trick-of-illusion). Dr Shastri in his writings on the Gītā often referred to these passages, as showing that the world is not evil, but a magic show put on by the Lord. True, there is a deception, but it is like the deception put on by actors in a classical drama, and voluntarily accepted by the audience, who feel the beauty in even tragic drama. However, their acceptance of the deception should not become involuntary: if it does, they will suffer. They must not give the stage show independent existence, so that they cannot dissolve its reality at will. They must see the Lord in all.

> On Me all this universe is strung,
> Like chains of pearls on a string.

The Gītā repeatedly states that these descriptions are to be taken as meditations; again and again it speaks of the yogin-devotee as 'yukta', which means literally 'yoked in yoga'. Yukta is in fact the same word as the English 'yoked'. Śaṅkara regularly glosses it as samādhi.

The chapters VII to X give warnings against taking the world as independently real, and against worship of some limited aspect of the Lord in order to get things desired. Such worshippers, if they have purity and faith, do indeed get what they have prayed for, though it may be only after a long time. It depends on the intensity and continuity of the prayer. But such selfish results can be only temporary, and they will have strengthened their own illusion.

Verses 16–18 give an early hint at the devotion of the one on the Path of Knowledge, who now seeks Freedom in the being of God:

VII.16 Four kinds of men worship Me, all virtuous people: those in distress, those seeking knowledge, those seeking success, and the Knowers.

17 Of them, the Knower, ever set in yoga with One-pointed devotion, is highest;
Very dear to the Knower am I, and he is dear to Me.

18 All of them are noble, but the Knower I take to be my very self; Firm in yoga he strives to reach Me, as the highest goal.

How is it that a Knower, who knows his Self to be the all-pervading creator-Lord already, can be said to strive to reach the Lord? This verse shows him striving, by yoga and devotion, to reach the Lord whom he already knows to be his own Self. It seems a contradiction, but this effort, this striving, is to remove memories of the past, which cloud his present direct awareness of identity. It is not to reinforce his Knowledge of the identity, which is an unshakable fact.

How is it that the fact seems to be shaken? Śaṅkara explains the point in detail in Chapter XIII, and elsewhere. For the moment it may be enough to recall that Napoleon, after he had become Emperor, was always rather nervous about his behaviour, though he knew that all he did would be accepted with fulsome praise. Similarly Nero, after becoming Emperor, was very nervous of failing in musical contests, though he knew that the judges would award him the victory. He knew, and yet memories of the past, before he was Emperor, somehow shook that knowledge, though they could never actually destroy it.

Chapter VIII Yoga-Power

Strength of Yoga

The practice of the eighth chapter presents mainly meditations on the Lord felt as within the body. First the mind and the prāṇa currents of vital energy are focussed at a centre in the heart. Then the focussed attention moves up with them to a point on the forehead roughly between the eyebrows. People who try this soon find that the concentration becomes confused. They are not sure when they have enough concentration to begin the move upward, and become indecisive.

The Gītā explains that it is done, and can only be done, by what it calls the 'strength of yoga'. Śaṅkara explains that this strength is in fact the after-effects of long practice, repeated till the saṃskāra-impressions have been formed strongly in the causal part at the root of the mind.

The process is then accomplished spontaneously, so to speak, independent of the discursive mind. Repeated practice has laid down impressions which now hold the samādhi completely steady.

It becomes a luminous movement, rising of itself, as it were. It is stronger than any interruption because the meditation is based on a natural current, latent in the ordinary man, but now showing itself. It is thus truth, and truth is stronger than the illusory concerns and memories of the world. But truth has to be brought out before it is experienced clearly.

The process can be seen in miniature in the drawing-up movement which occurs when any meditation, begun in a reasonable posture, begins to come to samādhi. There is usually the feeling of a current moving upward in the centre of the body. In some yoga systems it is called the 'upstroke'; Patañjali notes that it follows on prāṇāyāma practice, done for a certain time. The length of time to the first up-stroke is noted (counting in breaths). Then the process is repeated.

But formal prāṇāyāma practice is not an indispensible condition. Deep meditation alone can lead to it.

The Gītā refers to it as taking place even at the time of death, when worldy concerns might be expected to be at a peak.

Śaṅkara points out that normally this manifestation of the up-stroke would be the result of repeated practice during life, though it might also be from the direct grace of the Lord alone.

How is it practised? Some direct instructions are given by Swami Mangalnath in *The Heart of the Eastern Mystical Teaching*, a book by Dr Shastri, who had known Swami Mangalnath well:

> A few hints from my personal experience may perhaps be useful. The hollow in the centre of your body where the ribs join just below the breast bone is the best region on which to fix your mind in meditation. You may have heard the expression 'the lotus of the heart'; it refers to this point.

> You can apply a little sandal-paste to the spot and then concentrate your mind on it. Two hours a day is not too long a time for this practice. When you can fix your mind there at will, then visualize a lotus of bluish colour, and when this meditation is matured, 'imagine' an OM placed on the lotus, and meditate on it.

Often such a passage is read rather quickly. If interested, a reader will try to centre attention on the place in the breast, but it soon becomes vague, and then boring. He moves on to the lotus, and then the OM. He begins to get confused. Soon many other thoughts spring up in the mind. Why in the breast? he wonders. Why not in the forehead? And what exactly does a lotus look like? Soon the practice drops away. Occasionally he tries imagining the lotus flower in the breast but finds it is now mixed up with doubts and guesses, and finally random memories and ideas. He drops it, with the thought: 'I tried it, and it didn't suit me.'

How then is the practice done? It should be noted that Swami Mangalnath says: 'When you can fix your mind there at will.' There in the breast at will, only then visualize a lotus of bluish colour there. And when this meditation is matured, and only then imagine OM placed on the lotus, and meditate on it.

The exercise, then, is done step by step. One cannot rise to the next step till the foot is firmly planted on the present one. The spot is touched, and a little dab of perfume may be applied, to help the centring. Attention is brought back and back to the spot. It keeps running away, but if there is persistence for about three weeks, it remains for longer and longer periods. The practiser becomes aware of a sort of interior light there. He may also experience invigoration. He does not try to create such effects by auto-suggestion; in any case, when they happen, they are different from anything he could anticipate.

He may get a hint that the practice is developing on right lines when occasionally in the middle of the day, he feels spontaneously, without having thought of it, a little breath of peace in the heart. This is an indication that the saṃskāra-s are becoming stronger in the causal depths of the mind. Even at a time of great disturbance, perhaps temptations or fear, there will sometimes come this cooling breath from beyond. When such things begin to happen, it is time to go on to the next part of the practice: the visualization of the lotus.

Like all these visualizations, what is seen is not exactly what had been imagined as a lotus. But the description 'lotus' is enough to recognize the experience when it begins to manifest. In some schools there are descriptions of it as like a wheel, or like a shallow luminous bowl. As the saṃskāra-s are laid down, which conform to and reinforce the saṃskāra-s of location previously established, the state becomes vivid. It is an experience of something already there, not the actualization of the auto-suggestion. It is new, though recognizable from the meditation directions. Some of those who have had it say privately that the colour of the lotus is more beautiful than any colour they have ever seen. But limited beauty is not the aim of the practice, which must go on to transcendence.

The final step is to make out an OM, standing, so to say, on the lotus. The Sanskrit letter can be taken, or the printed Roman letters. These are forms representing the Word of Glory, the natural expression of the Lord. 'I am OM in the holy scriptures', 'Of expressions, I am that one syllable' (X.25). In this fundamental meditation, the form of the letters becomes sound and light.

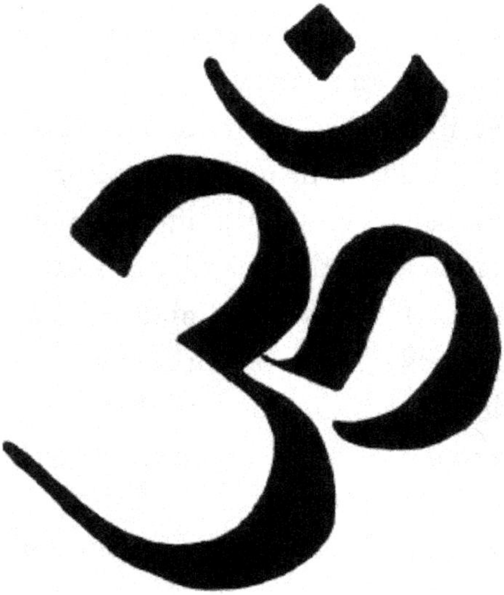

The holy syllable OM

This is one of the most direct ways of realizing the Lord as the Self: it requires determination, and detachment from worldly ties. Those who have been faced with a great tragedy are sometimes disillusioned for a time: and they have a good chance with this practice. It needs resolute application, and resolute independence. Swami Rama Tirtha made OM his main method for realization. He said, 'For one moment throw overboard all your attachments and anxieties, and chant OM. You will find yourself transformed into light.'

The final rise from the heart centre to the forehead centre is not the result of a conscious individual decision. If the basic yoga practice called the Line of Light, described here on page 205 has been carried out long enough for it to become natural, then the OM in the heart rises with the mind and prāṇa life-current. The yogin may be aware of it, or it may be as natural as digestion. It depends how much he has passed beyond personal restrictions. The blessing is the same. Though they often happen of themselves, the Gītā describes these things so that those yogins who do become aware of something happening do not become excited by it, or shrink back before the unknown. The Gītā description is enough for them to recognize it, and accept it.

Chapter IX and X Glories

In these two chapters, there is a flood of pictures for meditation and devotion. The aspects of the Lord are not restricted in time or place. There are some Indian references, but they are incidental; the main presentation is in terms of the whole world. This is not worship in a Kṛṣṇa cult. There are no accounts of incidents in the life of Kṛṣṇa as a personal avatar, such as are needed for the basis of a cult of one particular divine incarnation.

Important verses are IX.17 and 19:

> 17 I am the father of this world, the mother, the establisher, the grandsire,
> The aim of knowledge, the purifier, the syllable OM, and sacred hymns and chants.
>
> 19 I give heat, I hold back and send rains. Both immortality and death, the existent and non-existent, am I.

Verse IX.19 refers to the so-called laws of nature. It is an entirely unjustified assumption that they are largely mechanical, and that we already know all the main ones. The Gītā vision shows divine direction and supervision of the world-process. Verse 17 has declared that the ultimate purpose of the cosmic projection is love, like the love of parents. But that world-process includes the replacement of the old forms by new ones: I am immortality but also death.

In Chapter X are given meditations on the Lord as the best and highest in each class of beings. Of bodies of water, He is the ocean: of mountains, the Himalaya. Much of the list consists of allusions requiring a knowledge of Indian myths. (To give an idea of the poetical swing of the devotional verses of the original, I give now a few verses from Chapter IX of Sir Edwin Arnold's translation which he called *The Song Celestial*. The old English suits the subject here.)

I am the Sacrifice! I am the Prayer!
I am the Funeral-Cake set for the dead!
I am the healing herb! I am the ghee,
The Mantra, and the flame, and that which burns!
I am – of all this boundless Universe –
The Father, Mother, Ancestor, and Guard!
The end of Learning! That which purifies
In lustral water! I am OM! I am
Rig-Veda, Sama-Veda, Yajur-Ved;
The Way, the Fosterer, the Lord, the Judge,
The Witness; the Abode, the Refuge-House,
The Friend, the Fountain and the Sea of Life
Which sends, and swallows up; Treasure of Worlds
And Treasure-Chamber! Seed and Seed-Sower.
Whence endless harvests spring! Sun's heat is mine;
Heaven's rain is Mine to grant or to withhold;

Death am I, and Immortal Life I am,
Arjuna! SAT and ASAT, Visible Life,
And Life Invisible!

From Chapter X:

I am the Spirit seated deep in every creature's heart;
From Me they come; by Me they live; at My word they depart!

Vishnu of the Ādityas I am, those Lords of Light;
Marīchi of the Maruts, the Kings of Storm and Blight;

By day I gleam, the golden Sun of burning cloudless Noon;
By Night, amid the asterisms I glide, the dappled Moon!

Of Vedas I am Sāma-Ved, of gods in Indra's Heaven
Vāsava; of the faculties to living beings given
The mind which apprehends and thinks; of Rudras Śaṅkara.

But in one place the Lord says: 'Of the Vṛṣṇi clan, I am Vāsudeva; of the Pāṇḍava brothers, I am Dhanañjaya.' Vāsudeva is Kṛṣṇa himself, and Dhanañjaya is a familiar name for Arjuna as master archer. The supreme Lord who is proclaiming himself is now saying: 'I am You.' This is the highest declaration of Knowledge, but Arjuna makes no comment, here or later. He simply does not notice it. The instinct for preservation of individuality prevents him from taking it in, although he thinks, and later says, that he has understood it all – 'my delusion has vanished' (XI.1).

Arjuna is overwhelmed by the majesty and splendour of the revelations. He uses many terms of adoration, and not the familiar salutation 'Kṛṣṇa', as he asks to hear yet more of the glories, so that he can know the Lord in truth by meditating on them. This is a central point in the practice of karma-yoga: meditation on the Lord in glory is a direct means to knowledge of the Lord as the Self.

At the end of Chapter X he feels in ecstasy, and at the beginning of XI he asks to see directly – and without the process of meditation – the universal form of the Lord. He believes that all his delusions have gone, and that the vision will simply confirm for him the conceptions he has built up from what he has heard. But he does not realize what has been said. He must have smoothly accepted 'I am immortality, I am death' as a theoretical concept, for he made no reaction to it. He had not taken in what he heard, because he had not meditated upon it. He is going to have a shock.

Chapter XI Face to Face

The chapter begins with Arjuna's confident belief that his delusion has been dispelled. He has by now heard the supreme mystery of adhyātma, in the Lord's declarations of his own glories. Arjuna has forgotten that in Chapter VIII the adhāyatma was explained as the self-nature (sva-bhāva) in every man, not only the Lord outside. Again, he has heard the Lord say (X.20) 'I am the Self in the heart of all beings', but he could not incorporate that into his experience. There was an unspoken reservation: 'but not in *me.*' He could not apply the divine adhyātma glory to his own inner self. Similarly in II.17 it is said that the Self is everywhere: but in nearly all hearers there is an inner whisper: 'Yes, but not exactly *here.*'

Arjuna asks to see the universal form of the Lord directly. He assumes that what he will see will be somewhat as he has imagined it from the descriptions. The Lord gives him the divine sight which can see universal things; it is this same divine sight which Sañjaya the seer is using to witness and report the whole scene. These are not private trances, for both Arjuna and Sañjaya speak and move in the world while seeing the vision.

XI.7 Behold now the whole world of the moving and unmoving, united in my body;
And whatever else you may desire to see.

9 With these words, O king, the great Lord of yogic power
Showed to Arjuna his supernal form as Ruler God:

10 Of many mouths and eyes, of many wonderful forms,
With many marvellous ornaments, with many marvellous weapons poised,

11 Wearing marvellous garlands and garments with wonderful perfumes and unguents,
All wonderful, divine, infinite, facing all directions.

12 As if the light of a thousand suns should suddenly burst forth in the sky,
Such was the light of that supreme One.

13 Arjuna was beholding in the body of the God of Gods,
The whole world united, yet divided into many.

Arjuna cries out spontaneously in adoration:

18 You are the imperishable, the supreme One whom we seek; You are the ultimate support of this whole universe;
You are the immortal guardian of the eternal right;
I see that you are the everlasting Spirit.

The Lord now gives an additional grace to Arjuna: 'And behold whatever else you may desire to see', as he had just promised. The unspoken desire turns out to be the course and end of the coming battle. After the wonders of the main vision, the second part brings into focus the immediate future of Arjuna, his friends and his opponents. The future is partly determined and partly undetermined: for instance, the deaths of certain warriors are certain, but it is not certain who will kill them.

The vision becomes terrifying:

> XI.24 Touching the sky, aflame, of many colours, with yawning mouths and blazing enormous eyes,
> Truly, seeing you so, my inmost self is shaken, and I find no rest or peace, O Lord.
>
> 26 Into those mouths are rushing helplessly all the warriors and hosts of kings,
> Bhīṣma, Droṇa and that son of a charioteer too; And the chiefs of our own side likewise.

The Lord says:

> 32 I am time, poised to destroy and take away them all:
> Even without you, these warriors in their ranks shall all be killed.
>
> 33 So arise, win heroic glory, conquer the enemies and enjoy rulership.
> Already have they been slain, by Myself; do you be simply the instrument.

> 34 Droṇa and Bhīṣma and Jayadratha and Karṇa, and the other heroes,
> Do you slay. They are already slain by Me. Do not hesitate!
> Fight and conquer the enemy in battle.

Arjuna is aghast at this part of the vision. He had previously heard the Lord say, 'None but I am immortal Time' (X.33) and 'I am death that carries off all' (X.34), but when he sees Time engaged in killing those whom he knows well, he cannot bear it. He begs for the vision to be removed, and the Lord reappears in his familiar human form as the charioteer.

An important point is made here, by one of the Gītā master-strokes of insight. Sañjaya, the seer, is not emotionally shattered by the details of the vision, as is Arjuna the fighter. At the very end of the Gītā, Sañjaya says:

> As I recall again and again that most wondrous form of the Lord,
> Great is my amazement, and I thrill with joy again and again.

Sañjaya sees, and remembers, the universal vision with joy, because he is independent; Arjuna, as shown by his contemptuous reference to Karṇa as 'that son of the charioteer', is still caught up in the web of relationships.

Chapter XI ends with a verse which Śaṅkara says sums up the message of the Gītā, beginning with karma-yoga. The Lord speaks:

> 55 Doing My work, intent on Me, devoted to Me, free from attachment,
> Without hatred for any being – who is so, goes to Me.

The verse will be taken up immediately in the next chapter.

Chapter XII Devotion

This short chapter, which follows the overwhelming vision of the universal form, is important for practice. The Supreme, as Kṛṣṇa, answers Arjuna's question: is it better to practise yoga samādhi on the universal form, or on Self alone without attributes? Through the mouth of Kṛṣṇa, that Great Self replies that in general it is more feasible to meditate on form, that is on the Lord-with-attributes, because to meditate truly on the pure Self means dropping body-consciousness.

Many students of the Gītā, in the East and West, claim to take to the yoga of the attributeless, as based on pure Knowledge. They say that the Gītā itself places this higher, inasmuch as all forms of the Lord, like other forms, are associated with māyā, namely display-of-illusion. So worship and meditation on the Lord-with-attributes is in fact reinforcing illusion.

They do not usually realize that Identificative meditation on the absolute away from māyā must involve giving up also the māyā of individual body and individual mind. A modern teacher has remarked that when the meditation comes to this point, there is usually a sort of shrinking away in the face of what begins to look alarmingly like a void. That teacher added drily: 'It's no good promoting oneself to the sixth form before one can tackle the sixth-form syllabus.' Śaṅkara himself says that full worship-in-identity of the attributeless Brahman-Self is in general possible for Knowers alone; it becomes the process of their Jñāna-niṣṭhā or clearing residual memory-confusions from the face of Knowledge.

As to the karma-yoga samādhi practice, the Lord has in previous chapters given many different forms in which he is to be pictured and then realized: the brilliance in fire, the fragrance in earth, Vyāsa among the sages, the father and mother of the universe, the essence of every thing.

It is to be noted carefully that there is hardly any encouragement to meditate on the personal human form of Kṛṣṇa. 'Of the Vṛṣṇi clan I am Vāsudeva (Kṛṣṇa)' is on the same level with 'Vyāsa among the sages'. The whole emphasis is on the universal aspects.

Verses 6 and 7 give the peak of karma-yoga:

> XII.6 But for those who surrender all their actions before Me,
> Intent on Me, meditating on Me, worshipping in unwavering yoga,
>
> 7 I soon become the rescuer from the sea of endless birth and death,
> Of these whose thought is absorbed in Me.

Thus karma-yoga reaches its peak in samādhi on God, still taken as separate.

The next four verses give the typical Gītā method of Teaching Down, as applied to the karma-yogin's meditation on the Lord:

XII.8 Set your thought on Me alone, absorb your higher mind in Me;
You will finally come to abide in Me:
Do not doubt it.

9 But if you cannot remain steadily in samādhi on Me,
Then take to the yoga of regular practice as your means to reach Me.

10 If you do not succeed by that practice, then simply work for me; if you can do actions for My sake alone, then too you will attain perfection.

11 If you are not equal even to this, then practise yoga in giving up the fruits of all your actions, with mind subdued.

Śaṅkara strongly makes the point that it is not a question of comfortably ruling out the higher stages on the ground that one could not possibly do them. On the contrary, there are to be continual attempts at the higher stages; in so far as they fail, the lower ones are to be added. The lower ones are meant to lead to the higher realizations, which are never absolutely impossible, because they are reflections of the Lord already standing in the heart. The practiser must not fall into the idea of a ladder, in which a higher step cannot be reached till the foot is firmly planted on the one below it. The succession is only until Knowledge arises, which may happen at any stage. He says: Practising karma-yoga in giving up the fruits, you will attain purity of mind (sattva-śuddhi), then yoga-Samādhi, then Knowledge, and finally Release which is perfection.

Abandonment of the fruits of actions is no mere cliché; it can be done only by one who 'resorts to yoga, and who has subdued the mind'. Suppose one has been engaged in some socially valuable and long-worked-for project. Now that devoted worker sees it destroyed, by chance, or perhaps by malice. One who has not to some extent subdued the mind by yoga will hardly be able to feel calmly: 'I have worked hard, but I dedicated the outcome to the Lord; let it happen according to His will.' Most people would feel bitter, or resentful that the Lord had not done something to preserve this good work. As one hardworking devotee remarked frankly: 'I feel the Lord has rather let us down. I know His will must be done, but why does He will things like this?'

The constant references to dedicating the fruits of actions to the Lord, or casting all actions before the Lord or before Brahman, have to be understood in the light of the earlier description of karma-yogic action in Chapter II.48:

> Set in yoga do your actions, casting off attachment
> Be the same in success or failure; this being-the-same is called yoga.

Without the other limb of karma-yoga, namely meditation practice, inner serenity is hard to attain.

The chapter ends with eight beautiful verses describing one who is dear to God, and to whom God is dear. They speak of being silent and homeless, abandoning all undertakings, and ever in samādhi on the Lord. Śaṅkara takes the 'devotion to Me' as devotion of the man of Knowledge to the Self, in other words, jñāna-niṣṭhā.

The verses also speak of his being friendly and compassionate to all, so that the Gītā here, as elsewhere, sees the jñāna-niṣṭhā course as bringing welfare to the world. The eight verses should be compared with II.55–72. Another comparable passage is XIV.22–25, describing one who has transcended the guṇa-aspects of nature.

The Great Self speaks of the conduct of the Knower who is clearing away all memory-traces of not-Self:

> XII.13–20
> He who hates none, but is friendly and compassionate to all.
> Free from selfishness and I-ness, indifferent to pain and pleasure, patient,
>
> That yogin who is always content, whose self is firmly controlled,
> Whose mind and intellect are fixed on Me in devotion, he is dear to Me.
>
> Before whom the world does not tremble, and who does not tremble before the world;
> Free from thrill, haste, fear and fever, he is dear to Me.
>
> Unconcerned, pure, capable, indifferent, undisturbed,
> Abandoning all undertakings, in devotion to Me, he is dear to Me.
>
> Who neither delights nor loathes, neither grieves nor craves,
> Renouncing distinctions of good and evil, devoted to Me, is dear to Me.

The same to foe and friend, and in honour or disgrace,
The same in cold or heat, joy or sorrow, free from attachment,

To whom blame and praise are equal, speaking little, content with anything that comes,
Tied to no place, his mind set on truth, full of devotion, that man is dear to Me.

Those who revere this nectar of holy conduct here given,
Faithful, intent on Me, they are beyond measure dear to Me.

Chapter XIII The Field

Chapter XIII is said by Śaṅkara to be mainly a Knowledge-chapter. It begins with the knowledge of the Field (body, mind, also the deep causal layer that holds them together) and the Field-knower, which is the witness-consciousness that sees and is not affected or bound by what it sees. The Gītā itself states that this doctrine comes from the Upaniṣad-s: 'set out in the sūtra-s on Brahman, well reasoned and definite.' As in many Upaniṣad-s, the world is first taken as provisionally real, but ultimately with no independent existence of its own.

This chapter elaborates the brief description of the Self in Chapter II.

> II.17 But know: that is indestructible by which this all is pervaded;
> This imperishable one, nothing can destroy.
>
> 24 Neither can He be cut nor burnt, nor wetted nor dried;
> Eternal, present everywhere, fixed, immovable, everlasting is He.

> XII.25 Unmanifest is He, unthinkable is He,
> Unchangeable – so is He declared to be.

This had no effect then on Arjuna, who still felt himself an absolutely separate individual.

In Chapter XII the same Self spoke again through the mouth of the Lord:

> XII.3 But those who revere the Imperishable, the Indefinable, Unmanifest,
> Omnipresent and Unthinkable, the Immovable, Unchanging, Fixed,
>
> 4 Restraining the sense-currents, treating all alike, —
> They reach none but Me, delighting in the welfare of all beings.

The Self in both these places was spoken of as unthinkable; it is not an emptiness, which after all is definable. Again, it was said to be present everywhere, so some appearance of a world, a 'where', has been allowed. Now in this Chapter XIII, the Field, individual and cosmic both, is briefly described:

> XIII.5 The physical elements, I-ness, the higher mind (buddhi) and the unmanifest (causal),
> The ten senses plus one (lower mind), the five objects of the senses,
>
> 6 Desire, aversion, pleasure, pain, association, intellect, self-preservation –
> Such briefly is the Field with its modifications.

A crucial point, made several times already in the Gītā, is that mental faculties like 'I-ness', and activities like self-preservation, are part of the Field. They do not inhere in the Field-knower. There is often a tendency among modern readers to suppose that knowledge of the Self is somehow knowledge of an object, in other words, a mental operation. Provided external circumstances hold up reasonably well, the mental conviction 'I know the Self' can hold up too. But it is still something within the Field, and if the Field gets too disturbed, the seeming conviction may be shattered. After some such an experience, a would-be yogin can sometimes end up sceptical, even hostile to the whole idea of yoga.

The programme of the chapter is: (1) declaration of a Field-knower apart from Fields (verses 1 and 2); the Field-knower is also called Field-owner (verse 33); (2) a roughly ascending scale of spiritual practices ending with jñāna-niṣṭhā, clearing away the last obstructions to Self-knowledge; (3) declaration of the Universal Self, seemingly associated with but really free from, all worldly associations. So from verse 7 follows a list of twenty things to be practised, beginning with Humility. The Gītā calls them Knowledge. Śaṅkara points out that Humility itself cannot be equated with Knowledge: it is called Knowledge because it is a means to Knowledge. The first nine refer to behaviour in general:

> XIII.7 Humility, honesty, harmlessness, patience, uprightness, Service of a teacher, purity, firmness, self-control;

Then come qualities centred round detachment. It is to be noted that some aspirants may be in the householder role:

> 8 Turning away from sense objects, absence of egoism,

> Seeing clearly the painful restriction of birth, death, age, disease, and sorrow;
>
> XIII.9 Absence of attachment and clinging to sons, wife, property and the like:
> Constant evenness of mind in the face of events desirable or undesirable.

Now follows meditation, the immediate precursor of the rise of Knowledge:

> 10 Unwavering devotion to Me in single-minded yoga;
> Cultivation of solitude and distaste for society;

Verse 11, the last verse of the passage, shows that Knowledge having arisen must be steady, and that it has a goal, namely release.

> 11 Constancy in Knowledge of the Self,
> Keeping in view the purpose of that Knowledge of truth -
> The foregoing qualities are themselves called Knowledge: everything else is Ignorance.

The above list of twenty qualities, from Humility to Keeping in View the Purpose of Knowledge, is regarded by Śaṅkara as central. He quotes it in other major works, and here, in his summing up in the commentary to XVIII.55, he refers to it in the standard Sanskrit style as 'Humility and the others'. But to translate this as 'qualities like humility' is not faithful to his text or his thought. It means 'the twenty qualities beginning with Humility down to Keeping in View the Purpose of Knowledge of Truth.' The practice of the last two qualities is based on Knowledge, so that the whole group can be loosely called Knowledge.

The next section, verses 12–17, describes what is to be Known. It is the Self absolute, but includes the world-appearance manifested by the māyā trick-of-illusion. So there are apparent contradictions between the level of truth and the level of appearances, as there are contradictions between the world of the stage drama and the world of the actors who project it:

> XIII.12 I will declare what is to be known, whose Knowledge gives immortality:
> It is the beginningless supreme Brahman, definable neither as existent nor non-existent.
>
> 13 With hands and feet on all sides, and eyes, heads and mouths on all sides;
> With hearing everywhere, It stands unmoved, ever encompassing all.
>
> 14 Seeming to have sense qualities, yet free from all senses,
> Apart, yet supporting everything; free from guṇa-s, yet experiencing guṇa-s.
>
> 15 Outside of beings, and within them; unmoving, and yet moving;
> Subtle and so hard to realize; both far away and near It is.
>
> 16 Undivided, It stands seemingly divided in beings;
> It should be known as supporting the beings, and as their consumer and originator.

> XIII.17 Light of lights, It is said to be beyond darkness: Knowledge, the object of Knowledge, and the goal of Knowledge, It abides in the heart of all.

The contradictory statements bring out the illusory character of the world: 'unmoving, yet moving', 'apart, yet supporting everything'.

There is no direct connection between the world of Elsinore, and the world of the theatre which produces *Hamlet*. The theatre is not in the same world as the play, yet it supports it. The hero dies, yet does not die. The audience has come to appreciate the acting and suffer a little at the tragedy, yet not so much that it is taken as real. This is the knowledge on which the performance rests.

The Lord sums up in verse 18:

> Thus the Field, and also Knowledge, and the object of Knowledge have been briefly declared:
> My devotee, on realizing this, becomes what I am.

The final phrase, 'what I am', represents the Sanskrit mad-bhāvam, literally 'my being'. Both here and in other places in the Gītā, Dr Shastri translated this as 'what I am'. This follows Śaṅkara's strong assertion that the essence of the individual self is the supreme Lord, 'as is so clearly taught in the Gītā and all the Upaniṣad-s'.

After this declaration of the final truth, and the means to it, the Gītā comes down to a lower level for those who cannot manage to incorporate it into their experience. It provisionally allows the reality of what happens in the world: Puruṣa the spirit is entangled in Nature, the Field-knower is caught up into attachment for the Field which he experiences.

XIII.21 The spirit, standing in Nature, experiences the guṇa-s born of Nature;
Attachment to the guṇa-s causes his birth into good and evil wombs.

This lower truth is presented by the Gītā in the technical concepts and terms of an early school; for the reader today, there is no advantage in analysing them. It is temporarily accepted that the experiences, and the attachment, really happen; the way out of them is purification of the basis of the mind by meditation, deep introspection, yogic action without making claims on the results, hearing the truth with reverence. Such actions lead to vision of the all-pervading Lord.

27 He sees, who sees the supreme Lord standing equally in all beings,
The undying in the dying.

28 For seeing the same Lord established in all,
He kills not the Self by the self; then he goes to the highest goal.

When the Lord becomes apparent as his own Self, and also apparent in the seeming others, then that individual body-mind Field will never impede the progress towards Self-realization of others. That would be to kill the Self in them, though only for a time it is true.

The chapter returns to the higher truth that there is no real entanglement of the Self in Nature; it only seems to be located in a body because of its manifestation there. Śaṅkara gives the example of the moon, which when reflected in puddles seems to be divided, located in many places, and dirty or actively disturbed according to the condition of the puddle surface. In fact none of these things is true of the moon.

> XIII.31 This supreme imperishable Self, beginningless and free from guṇa-s,
> Even abiding in the body, neither acts nor is tainted.
>
> 33 As the sun, shining alone, illumines the whole world,
> So the Field-owner illumines the whole Field.
>
> 34 Those who with the eye of Knowledge can distinguish the Knower from its Field.
> And realize freedom from Nature – they go to the highest.

At the end of this chapter on Knowledge, it must be recalled that the pure Knowledge is not an idea. Ideas are the business of the Field, not of the Field-knower. The pure focussed mind gets glimpses of the reflection of the sun of the Field-knower, but in final liberation mind is absorbed in the sun. It is Being absolute, and not knowledge of an object.

Looking steadily into themselves with the 'eye of Knowledge' in the stillness of focussed meditation on the truths of the teaching, they dimly make out something unmoving in the moving mind, something undying in the ever-dying thoughts and experiences, something infinite in the apparent restrictions. If this is not disturbed by the restless wavering mind which tries to preserve its limited interests, the horizons of freedom open out.

Chapter XIV The Guṇa-s

The doctrine of the three guṇa-s or basic elements of the cosmos is presented in the Gītā. It is not a central Upaniṣadic doctrine. The Gītā prescribes a knowledge of them as an aid to practice in daily life. The treatment is mainly in Chapters XIV and XVII, with a group of verses in Chapter XVIII.

Chapter XIV in fact begins with one of the analogies of the world-process, which come in several places in the Gītā. It is represented in terms of fertilization of Nature by the Lord. A major point of the analogies is, that the world-appearance is a conscious divine projection; delusive and a source of suffering when not recognized as such, it is bliss when realized as the Lord. The Lord must be realized not only externally, but as the Self, the Knower of the Field. Each analogy is intended as a stimulus to experience; they are not mutually consistent in details, though they are often introduced as a great 'secret'. As was pointed out in the section on Teaching Down, each successive revelation is for some people the final clue or 'secret' which makes all clear. Only in so far as they do not 'see and know', is further instruction needed.

The word 'guṇa' meant originally the strand of a rope, but soon came to be used for an attribute, especially a good attribute. But the sense of an actual thing or element was not lost. Guṇa-s are the fundamental constituents of the cosmic manifestation, and as such have phases: physical, mental, and causal. There are three of them: sattva, goodness, relative truth, and by extension, light, purity, balance and calm; rajas, passion-struggle, and by extension selfishness and pain; tamas, darkness, and by extension inertia and delusion. The three bind the embodied self, by their respective forces of attachment:

> XIV.6 Sattva, pure, illuminating, and healthy
> Yet binds by attachment to happiness and by attachment to knowledge.
>
> 7 Know that rajas, whose nature is to desire because of thirst and clutching attachment,
> Binds the embodied by attachment to action.
>
> 8 Know that darkness of tamas, arising from ignorance, deludes all the embodied,
> Binding them by heedlessness, laziness and sleep.

Even sattva is a binding force, though the bonds are light; they are silver chains which can be taken as prestige symbols in life. Even the purest sattva is part of the Field, and it binds (or, as Śaṅkara adds, appears to bind) the Self in a particular Field.

The guṇa-s are all present all the time in the whole of Nature, including of course the Field. A yogin's life is predominantly sattvic, but still his body or mind sometimes feels slack or restless. He can modify these impulses. In the ordinary way, tamas is overcome by rajas, and then rajas has to be purified and calmed by sattva. Sattva does not so easily influence tamas directly. At the outset of the Gītā, it is by rajas that the Lord rouses Arjuna out of complete tamas; he brings forward frankly rajasic considerations, of honour and disgrace and so on. Arjuna is roused from the inert 'I will not fight' of II.9 to at least listening to the teaching, and so to the 'What shall I do?' of III.2. He had said this earlier on, but it was swept aside by 'I will not fight'. This time he is beginning to mean it.

The habitually dominant guṇa-attitude during life will determine the state at death, and some of the conditions of future lives. Some account of this is given in the Gītā. But in the West, where reincarnation is merely a hypothesis, such passages are often a distraction. They can lead to fruitless discussions for or against. When yoga practice advances, there may be experiences which settle the matter for the individual. Śaṅkara confirms this. But in general, the stress in the Gītā is on attainment of freedom in this very life. It is the guṇa-s that bind, or seem to bind; they are to be transcended either by Knowledge, as in II.45 and XIV.19, or by devotion and service of the Lord as in XIV.26.

> 19 When the Seer sees no other agent than the guṇa-s
> And knows the higher-than-the-guṇas, he becomes what I am.

Towards the end of XIV, Arjuna asks one of his questions, this time about the marks of the one who has gone beyond the guṇa-s. It shows that he does not yet have much idea of the Self free from all attributes; any marks could apply only to the purified

Field, from which the feeling of self is now withdrawn. The Lord answers the question in the terms in which it has been put. He gives the main characteristics of the body-mind complex which is practising jñāna-niṣṭhā; they are mainly negative:

> XIV.24 to whom loved and unloved are equal, to whom blame and praise are equal... alike to friend and foe,... to whom pain and pleasure are alike, abiding in the self, to whom clods, stones and gold are all one;
>
> 25 abandoning all undertakings...

Most of them have been given in the Knowledge-yoga sections at the end of II, the end of XII, and elsewhere; 'to whom clods, stones and gold are all one' comes also in VI.8; 'abandoning all undertakings' was one of the qualities listed in XII. 16.

Important for practice is a new theme:

> XIV.22 Light (i.e. sattva), activity (rajas), and delusion (tamas), arising in him,
> He does not hate when they come, not long for them when they have ceased.

This can be misunderstood as a sort of fatalism. But that is against the clear words of the verse. The yogin takes energetic action to remove tamas in his mind, for instance by study or service; he calms the disturbance of rajas by meditation. But he does not hate rajas and tamas: he just removes them. Nor does he long for sattva when it is temporarily absent: 'Oh, alas! I have fallen away from the state of purity.' He simply restores it, without getting excited. In the same way, on a cold morning a musician knows that his hands will be slow and imprecise. But he does not curse the weather, or long for it to change. He knows that it will take more of the usual exercises to warm up the hands, and he calmly does them. Profound is the meaning of a Japanese Zen poem:

> Every day we sweep up the fallen leaves in the garden;
> But we do not hate the trees for dropping them.

The Gītā sets out the effects of the guṇa-s on human personality and action. The sattvic agent is detached, non-egoistic, firm and vigorous, but unaffected in success or failure. The rajasic agent is passionate, greedy, cruel, impure, and elated or depressed according to how things turn out. Dominated by tamas, he is unreliable, crude in his methods, unteachably obstinate, sly, wicked, lazy and easily discouraged.

Main points are summarized in the chart in Chapter XVII on page 155. To read the chart horizontally gives the different phases, with a view to recognizing the present phase, and bringing it ultimately to sattva. To read vertically gives unalloyed pictures of the predominance of sattva, or rajas, or tamas.

Some of the points of the analysis are subtle. The action of rajas is said to be 'with tiring effort'. This means that things are forced through, by employing means against the nature of the situation. On a small scale, this would cover gripping the pen very tightly, or banging the keys of a typewriter. There is no love for the nature of the instruments used.

Again, the firmness of tamas is said to be that by which a dull person holds fast to fear and grief. At first sight, this can seem surprising, but the Gītā is pointing out how neurosis protects itself: it is somehow 'me', as some sufferers frankly admit. Then those who practise 'terrifying austerities', with self-torture, are said to be imbued with the strength of lust; thus the Gītā discourages such feats as sexual perversions.

Reading down the column of sattva, some feel a distaste for the repeated phrase 'it is to be done', 'it is to be sacrificed', 'it is to be given'. They feel that it is compulsive morality, lacking in the human feeling which should be the basis of action. There is an echo of a tight-lipped character in Ibsen, saying coldly, 'It was my duty, and I did it,' clearly without much pleasure. The advocates of 'human feelings' believe in a gift from a spontaneous uprush of sympathy.

That is not the Gītā basis for gift or action. The analysis is profound. Gifts can be made from a rush of feeling, but feelings are of many kinds. A feeling of love for some unfortunates often leads to hatred of those who are regarded as their oppressors. Marx's idealism soon led him to destructive hatred of the capitalist class: he hated them even though on his own reasoning they were bound to behave as he predicted. On this point, Marx's opponent, the anarchist Bakunin, saw more clearly: 'Put peasants where the nobles now are, and they will behave exactly as the nobles are doing.'

To feed the starving in a famine-stricken village in a remote, cut-off country must be good, but if done simply from sympathy it may lead to agonizing decisions. The amount of food is limited: is it better to share it out evenly, in which case everyone will die before the next harvest anyway; or is it better to let some die now, and give the relatively strong all the food, to keep them going and working till they can get the next harvest in?

Sometimes midwives in primitive communities have been shown simple means of saving some babies who otherwise died: but those children died of starvation after a very few years, because there was not enough food to support an increase in population.

Again, some tribes are marauders, practising skill with weapons, and living by plunder. In one famine, when the United Nations relief convoys came, the tribes who worked the land begged them not to feed the equally starving robber tribe. 'When they get strong again, they'll come down at the next harvest time and plunder our grain stocks. They kill any of us who resist.' The relief convoy did in fact distribute food to all, but one of them said afterwards: 'I am haunted by the uncertainty whether we did right or not.'

The Gītā teaching on this point would say that such a gift would not be 'to a worthy person', and would not be a yogic gift. It could still be given, but it would not contribute to the ultimate welfare of the world. Looking at the pathetically starving marauders, fellow-feeling will say; 'Give!' Looking at the graves of those whom they recently killed, fellow-feeling will say: 'Don't set these killers up again!'

The Gītā itself says:

> XVIII.48 One should not give up the action proper to one's role, though it may have some bad effects,
> For all actions have something defective in them, as a fire has smoke.

The dilemma in hoping to do unqualified good is summed up by an Eastern poet: He who is kind to tigers is a tyrant to sheep.

Until the inner instruments are so purified that the divine impulse flows through them, totally devoid of individual self-reference, actions have to be governed by tradition as laid down in the great scriptures. Control of the mind has to be practised, so that there is no elation or depression at results, nor picking and choosing to follow only self-selected rules of conduct.

> XVI.23 Those who disregard the injunctions of the divine Law and live according to their own wilful desires,
> Do not attain perfection, nor bliss, nor the supreme goal.
>
> 24 Therefore let the injunctions of the Law be your authority
> In determining what should and should not be done.
>
> XVIII.9 When such required action is done simply because it ought to be done,
> Abandoning attachment to it, and also to the fruit of it -
> That abandonment is said to be of sattva.
>
> 10 The man of sattva who has thus abandoned attachment is wise and has no doubts:
> He does not recoil from unpleasant action (when righteousness demands it), nor does he cling to an agreeable one.

Sattva leads to happiness, rajas leads to pain, tamas to delusion. Happiness arises when the mind becomes serene. To attain serenity of mind requires effort at detachment, distinguishing what is real from what is not, and especially practice of meditation (dhyāna) and samādhi. Strong and persistent efforts have to be made. The Gītā humorously compares them to 'poison at first', leading to inner peace which is 'nectar in the end'.

> XVIII.37 The happiness of sattva is said to be like poison at first and nectar when it develops;
> Arising from serenity of the mind (reflecting) the inner Self.

There is a momentary experience of happiness when some strong rajasic desire has just been fulfilled. The happiness in fact does not arise from the fulfilment, for repetition often yields less and less happiness from it. The happiness comes from the temporary peace and stillness of the mind. The desire had become the whole world; the other considerations of the world had for the time being vanished. So on fulfilment there is a feeling that everything has been done, everything has been successful, everything has been fulfilled. There is a stillness; other desires have vanished. But very soon they return: fears, jealousies, ambitions, tense expectations, return with greater force because they have been neglected.

> XVIII.38 The happiness of rajas is declared to be like nectar at first and poison as it develops,
> Arising as it does from attaining union with some object of the world.

The happiness of tamas is silliness and delusion from beginning to end: it has been compared by a Japanese Buddhist to the happiness of a man drunk in a night-club on a fake expense account. It does not last long.

This Japanese was a famous counsellor, whose recommendations were supported by some wealthy charitable men. His spiritual advice, often very short, had saved a number from suicide. He remarked that though the physical wants could be met a little, the mental sufferings were often worse.

He added that there is little genuine happiness in the mere fact of trying to do good: the one who does good is by that very fact in a superior position, and any supposed happiness is often disguised self-congratulation, or even domination. It has a reaction. 'Confronted all day with endless misery, I knew that what I can do of myself is little enough. Only when I feel the Buddha's hands moving in my hands, the Buddha's speech behind anything I might say, is there real happiness.'

Mother Teresa of Calcutta has commented about social work without a religious basis: 'It is very good, but it is not the work of Christ. To do the work of Christ, there must be love of silent contemplation in solitude.'

Rajas in the form of desire to dominate is always seeking to take over undertakings that began as sattva. Without meditation, it is not easy to recognize. But through meditation:

> XI.55 Doing My work, intent on Me, devoted to Me, free from attachment,
> Without hatred for any being – who is so, goes to Me.

Chapter XV One and Many

Chapter XV is a summary presentation of the Gītā teachings, as the chapter itself declares in the last verse. It is also one of the shortest chapters, only twenty verses. Anyone who seriously intends to practise the yoga of the Gītā must learn some central part of it by heart, in order to get some inner resources to meet difficult or bewildering situations. The twenty verses of XV make a firm basis for practice.

It begins with one of the analogies of the world-process, this time as a tree. The analogy of the sacred fig-tree, called in Sanskrit aśvatta, like others in the Gītā, is taken from an Upaniṣad. This time it is the Kaṭha Upaniṣad, VI.1. The Lord has already said in Gītā X.26: Among all the trees, I am the sacred aśvattha.

The symbolic tree has its main root in heaven, showing that the world-process is divine in origin. In a living tree, every part is connected with every other part, and this illustrates that the world is an integrated whole. It is, however, a divinely projected illusion, and those who are caught by the belief in its independent reality must cut that down.

XV.1 They tell of the eternal fig-tree, with root above and branches below.
Its leaves are the Vedic hymns; he who knows the truth of it, knows the Veda.

2 Down and up stretch its branches, nourished by the guṇa-s, and budding out into sense-objects,
Below also stretch forth its secondary roots, resulting in human worldly action.

3 It is not known as such in this world, neither its end nor origin nor basis.
Let one cut down this firmly rooted tree with the stout axe of non-attachment, -

4 And seek out that realm from which no one is forced to return
(Meditating) 'I resort to that very primal spirit from whom first streamed forth the ancient current.'

As will be shown, this seeking for the unchanging realm, this resorting to the eternal Spirit, is not a question of believing in something in the distant past, or praying to a remote deity now. The realm of immortality, and the eternal Spirit, are behind present human experience of constant change. One way to seek the Spirit which is the root of the magic tree is to sit still, and try to isolate the source of the magic tree of our many-branched thoughts. Without some such yogic practice, as verse 11 will declare, it is not possible to detect him, however much one may believe in and study the holy texts.

5 With no pride or delusion, with attachment conquered, steady in the Self, desires cast off,
Free from pleasure and pain, clear-sighted men go to that eternal place.

6 That needs no sun to light it, nor moon nor fire;
From which none has to return, – that is my supreme state.

In 5 and 6, the Lord has spoken of how to reach the state of transcendence, one with the Lord in his supreme state. But as so often, the Gītā proclaims that the Supreme can also be known in the illusions of māyā. In māyā, the Lord is apparently limited and separated off by body, senses and mind, and karmic connections. The Lord becomes many, and is confused, and broken up, by events of the world. Śaṅkara illustrates this by the example of the one sun which is reflected in many puddles; it becomes many, and is sometimes serene, sometimes thrown into waves, and sometimes broken up into disordered fragments, all according to the passing changes in the water of the puddles. Yet one who has the 'eye of Knowledge' sees the sun above, and knows the states of the reflected suns for what they are. Then he can enjoy them.

7 It is a ray of mine alone which in this world becomes the ever-persisting individual soul;
It draws to itself from Nature the senses, with the mind as the sixth.

8 When He takes up a body, and again when He leaves it, the Lord moves taking them with Him,
As the wind takes perfume from flowers.

9 Using hearing, sight and touch, taste and smell,
And the mind, he absorbs himself in objects of sense.

10 Deluded men do not see Him, surrounded by the guṇa-s,
when He goes, or stays, or experiences objects;
Those who have the eye of knowledge, see Him.

11 The yogin-s, sincerely striving, see Him there in the self;
But those who have not thus trained themselves, do not see
Him however much they try, dulled as they are.

The strong efforts of the yogin-s are needed, adds Śaṅkara, to get rid of the obstacles to vision of the Self. The vision does not need strengthening or reinforcing; it is a present fact. Under the light of the Self, indeed, the obstacles themselves are perceived as existing independently. They are illusory, but powerful when taken to be self-existent.

What sort of efforts are needed? Imagine a girl brought up since childhood under a dictatorship. She has been told never, never to speak of anything to do with even local government. She has been frightened by stories of terrible unspecified things that can happen to free speakers. Now she comes to the free society, where she hears and sees people making furious criticisms of official actions or lack of them. She is asked for her opinion on the desirability of a pedestrian crossing near her home, but avoids answering. She tells her friends: 'I know it would be all right to speak, but somehow I can't. I daren't'. A good friend runs over the clear facts with her, but it has no effect. So the friend says: 'Well, as an exercise, try speaking these words: "They ought to put a crossing there."' She does it, but cannot stop her voice from trembling. So now the friend allows a sort of provisional reality to her fears, and says: 'Try reading this critical newspaper editorial aloud to me, in a corner. After all, they are not your words. So you needn't feel guilty.' She just manages this. After a few days, in which nothing happens: 'Now try reading it aloud to a group of us.' A little more confident this time. 'Now try saying it in your own words.' Still better. 'Good. You are free, you know, free. Now say something of your own, about something you don't agree with.' In this way, by patient efforts which involve courage and resolution, the illusion is dissolved. Provisionally taken as real, it is step by step dissipated. But the steps do not correspond to any external reality; the friend must add from time to time: 'You are quite free, you know, quite free.' Otherwise shreds of illusion may remain, such as that it is only safe to quote a newspaper, or to speak in a corner, and so on.

Now the Lord declares some of the manifestations in which he can be seen most easily:

> 12 The splendour of the sun which illuminates the whole world, and that in the moon and in fire,
> Know that to be My splendour.
>
> 13 Entering into the earth, I support all beings by its strength,
> And I nourish all plants as their sacred essence.
>
> 14 Becoming the fire set in the body of living beings,
> I join with the ascending and descending vital currents,
> And digest their food of various kinds.

> 15 I have entered into the heart of all; from Me come memory, knowledge and their loss.
> I alone am to be known from all the Vedas, and I am the author of the Upaniṣad-s and their knower.

The examples given of the divine manifestations are indications for realization practice; they are not meant to be exclusive. The Lord is more easily seen in the splendour of the sun than in a brick wall, says Śaṅkara: but he is equally present. We recognize the same principle in teaching science: the action of gravity is more easily recognized with small weights dropping in a vacuum than in dried leaves blown about by an autumn gale. But the principle of gravity is equally operative.

'I have entered into the heart of all': this is a central principle of yoga metaphysics. 'From Me come memory, knowledge and their loss': in accordance with past actions of each being in this and previous lives. Memory and knowledge of spiritual truth come from good karma; their loss comes from bad karma. It is the Lord who joins the cause to the corresponding effect. However, karmic conditions are not absolutely determined and unalterable, since there is always an indefinite amount of unfulfilled past karma from the beginningless series of past lives. There must have been some good actions in those lives, because with the alternation of the guṇa-s, sometimes sattva is dominant. And in this birth too there are moments of clarity in even the most disturbed and darkened life. Such moments may be very short. If the chance is grasped, the present karma can be modified, especially by recognition of the Lord's hand in it, and his friendliness to all beings. If He is concentrated on, and worshipped, as the friend of all beings (V.29), even difficult circumstances will be adjusted (not necessary completely removed) to provide spiritual opportunities.

> XV.16 Here in this world are two spiritual principles: the perishable, and the imperishable;
> The perishable is all beings; the imperishable is the unmoving, the illusion on which they stand.
>
> 17 But there is a highest spirit, beyond, which is called the supreme Self;
> It is the undying Lord who enters and supports the three worlds.
>
> 18 Since I transcend the perishable, and am higher than even the imperishable,
> By worldly thinkers and in the scriptures, I am proclaimed to be the highest spirit.

Verse 16 can be a surprise. The very words 'imperishable' and 'unmoving', which have been repeatedly used for the supreme Spirit, are here demoted, as it were, to apply to the cosmic trick-of-illusion which the Gītā elsewhere calls māyā. Formally it is a contradiction, but it has an important meaning for practice. Words used to point to the transcendent tend gradually to become assimilated to this world. Their provisional nature is forgotten, and they come to represent *things*. For example, the Lord is taken as more and more human; he is thought to become angry, jealous, partial, or arbitrary. Human-type reasons are proposed for his creation of the universe; human-type criticisms are made for his supposed wastefulness in creating uninhabited galaxies as a background to the human drama. Words like imperishable, unmanifest, or unchanging become peripheral attributes of an omnipotent but somewhat capricious deity.

The Gītā repeatedly cautions against the tendency. Along with positive descriptions like all-pervading, it uses words like 'unthinkable', 'indefinable'; in a main passage on Brahman (XIII.12) it says: 'It cannot be said to be.' In these ways, again and again it warns against taking the Absolute as a *thing*. The indications are not anything more than pointers; this is one reason why they are sometimes contradicted after having been given. The Lord is called 'unmanifest', but in VIII.18 and 20 unmanifest is lowered in meaning so that it indicates the mayic source of all beings, while the Lord is 'more unmanifest than the unmanifest'.

In view of the danger of taking words as realities, it might be wondered why they are used at all. Some spiritual teachers have indeed largely rejected words. In one tradition Bodhidharma, who carried Zen Buddhism to China, would not explain in words. The disciple meditated and periodically put forward his view, to which Bodhidharma replied only: 'No, No!' This follows the recommendation of one Upaniṣad: 'Few words need be used.' (Muṇḍaka 2.2.5)

But the Gītā believes that for a time words are most useful, in spite of the danger that they will become a substitute for realization. Words like 'imperishable' are to be meditated on, and will lead to a flash of awareness of immortality in the meditator, but not if they become conceptual counters in an intellectual game. The signpost, though marked 'LONDON', does not mean this is London itself.

19 He who, undeluded, knows Me thus as the supreme Spirit, He knows everything, and worships Me with his whole being.

20 This most secret teaching has been declared by Me; One awakened to this, would be truly awakened, and would have done all that he had to do.

To know, without delusion, the Lord as the highest spirit, who has entered and who supports the three worlds, is to awaken to: 'I am He.' Before this awakening the Lord is believed to be all-pervading, as the text says, but there is an unspoken qualification: 'but not here, and not in me.' When the awakening comes, the remaining thin bonds of restriction to the body-mind complex are dissolved.

What then does it mean to say that he knows everything, and that he worships? There is no separate-seeming self; only the Lord is there, within and without. He, the Lord, knows everything in the sense that he is everything. God does not think or know as a mental operation: there is nothing apart, nothing separate, for him to know as an object. But the surviving body-mind complex, though a mere shadow, can still be referred to as 'he'; this it is which carries on the jñāna-niṣṭhā, divinely inspired and delighting in the welfare of all beings, till its illusory separate existence finally fades away into light.

Chapter XVI Passion-Struggle

The chapter begins with a list of things innate in those in whom the impulse towards liberation is becoming strong: they are said to be of divine nature. Those who fear it, cling to their own individuality and hate competing individualities, are of demoniac nature.

The chart below sets out the present list, alongside XIII.7–10 (qualities to be cultivated by a seeker of Knowledge), and the programme of Austerity in XVII, and XVIII 42–14 which identifies actions 'natural' to Brahmins, warriors, businessmen, and men of service.

Many of them appear in more than one list; for instance, dhṛti or firmness is said to be natural to a warrior; nevertheless XIII says it is to be cultivated by Knowledge-seekers, and by all who desire liberation, according to XVI. It is clear that these 'innate' qualities, or actions as they are called in XVIII, are not self-sufficient. Compare a talent for music, which has to be arduously developed if it is to show its full capacity.

Qualities to be cultivated by karma-yogin-s, listed by Chapters

	XVI	**XVII**	**XVIII**	**Leading to Knowledge, Chapter XIII**
	(occurring in all four lists)			
self-control	○	○	Brahmin	•
uprightness	○	○	Brahmin	•
purity	○	○	Brahmin	•
	(occurring in three lists)			
devotion-worship	○	○		•
steady yoga	○		Brahmin	•
gift	○	○	Kṣatriya	
tapas	○	○	Brahmin	
serenity	○	○	Brahmin	
firmness	○		Kṣatriya	•
non-violence	○	○		•
	(occurring in two lists)			
fearlessness	○		Kṣatriya	
purity of essence	○	○		
self-study	○	○		
truth	○	○		
giving up fruits	○	○		
fire	○		Kṣatriya	
patience	○		Brahmin	
service			Śūdra	•
no pride	○			•
	(occurring in one list)			
sincerity				•
non-egoity				•
realization: all is pain				•
withdrawal				•
non-attachment				•
undisturbability				•

	XVI	XVII	XVIII	Leading to Knowledge, Chapter XIII
yoga meditation on God				•
solitude				•
steadiness in self-Knowledge				•
freedom as goal				•
no anger	○			
no slander	○			
compassion	○			
no craving	○			
gentleness	○			
modesty	○			
no fickleness	○			
not injuring	○			
brahmacarya (chastity)		○		
true and beneficial speech		○		
charm		○		
faith		○		
silence		○		
authority			Kṣatriya	
skill			Kṣatriya	
heroism			Kṣatriya	
belief			Brahmin	

There are three which appear in all four lists: self-control, uprightness and purity. Seven appear in three lists: worship, steady yoga, gift, austerity (which covers a very wide field of conduct), peace, firmness, non-violence. Often the Sanskrit word is exactly the same. (There are some fine distinctions which are irrelevant for practice.)

Some critics point to what they call the negative nature of the lists. Of the ten qualities just mentioned, Giving would be (they say) the only positive act of benevolence. The Gītā view is that most material sufferings could be fairly easily remedied if the basic nature of those concerned were purified. Famines caused by natural disasters are quickly relieved by national or international co-operation. But famines caused by civil or other wars (the vast majority) go on and on; gifts of food from outside are only palliative. The Gītā does not agree with the comment of Karl Marx: 'The philosophers have only interpreted the world in various ways: the point is, to change it.' Yoga would say: 'The philosophers have only interpreted human nature in various ways: the point is, to change it.' The objection that human nature cannot be changed is patently untrue: there are, and always have been, regions of the world where the natural fear and hate of strangers have been replaced by consideration and care for them. In India in 300 BC there were special courts to protect them from being exploited.

The morality of the Gītā, as shown here and elsewhere, is not compulsive in the sense of against nature. The qualities and virtues are 'innate'; they have to be cultivated, but this is 'following the stream', as it is said. Those who act and think in a contrary way are going against their own deeper nature. They suffer accordingly till they change the flow back to what it should be by nature.

Important is the example given by those who demonstrate freedom from selfish or trivial considerations. The conduct of those who are looked up to as spiritually great will be followed, to some extent at least, by others. It is a fact that simply to see someone free from personal motives is a stimulus to try for freedom; it activates the innate tendency towards freedom in those who are beginning to awaken.

Most of the rest of the chapter describes those of demoniac nature, to whom anger and cruelty seem like justifiable indignation. To dominate is to them a natural goal: the world is for the strong or cunning. It has no creator, or integrating principle: it is simply here, and to think about it is meaningless. What matters is to fulfill one's desires, especially for 'greatness'. The Gītā shows how they are endlessly led on by fantasies of glory. A modern yogin has remarked: 'This attitude is never satisfied with mere success: it wants a Roman triumph. And it spends more energy, and takes greater risks, to get that triumph than just to succeed.'

In fact such men and women, dominating others, are themselves dominated by endless anxieties and fears. They come to live, says the Gītā, in a foul hell. The text says that they hate the Lord in themselves and in others. There is a half-unconscious fear of the divine element. As a result they never come to know the Lord. This 'never' is simply a strong assertion of difficulty: the Gītā itself has said in VI.36 that even the worst of such sinners can cross beyond the sea of evils by Knowledge, and in IX.31 that even a very evil-doer can be quickly saved by the grace of the Lord.

The guṇa-s alternate, though one is habitually predominant in an individual. Even in the most sinful and deluded, sunk in rajas and tamas, there are moments, usually very short, of pure sattva, when the vision becomes clear. (It is the mirror image of the case where a saint is suddenly assailed by an impulse of passion.) If in that brief moment of sattva he can look unflinchingly towards the Self, or can turn resolutely to the Lord with his whole being, then the radical transformation takes place. 'But,' as an experienced yogin remarked, 'usually people are so identified with their own past and present that they feel such a complete change would kill them.'

The chapter ends with the instruction to follow traditional authority as to what to do and what not to do. The holy texts of revelation give general guides to conduct. Such authority can be compared to the rules of grammar. They have to be followed in the main, in order to communicate the meaning. An expert writer can break the rules to get a particular effect, but he does not break them much. A beginner who tries to imitate this freedom simply becomes incomprehensible. In the same way, to argue with a passion-dominated mind against tradition, because it is felt to be restrictive, is self-defeating. The traditions correspond to depths in man which may be quite unsuspected. Practice of the tradition will bring out flowers, and powers, from those depths. But when divine inspiration comes through a purified and clear mind, rules are no longer necessary.

Faith

XVII.2 Deep-seated in the nature of man is faith, which is threefold: of the nature of Light (sattva), of Passion-struggle (rajas) and of Darkness (tamas).
3 A man is what his faith is. As his faith is, so is he, undoubtedly.

Dr Shastri says: 'This chapter starts with a description of the basic tendency in the nature of each individual, which gives rise to, and colours, his thought and action. Our mental, emotional and physical activities are actuated by this deep mystic tendency which is called Faith. It is the aggregate of the subtle impressions left by our past lives on our causal body. Man can create, control and change this tendency; it is not an unalterable fate.'

The 'subtle impression' is what is technically called 'saṃskāra'. We are familiar with this in ordinary life. If we touch an electrical appliance and get a shock, we thereafter approach them with caution. If, in spite of this, we happen to get another shock from one, we may come to fear them unreasonably.

Such impressions can be constructive also. We gradually get to know the gears of a car, by repeated use, until handling them is almost automatic. We should note that skills are laid down at the beginning consciously, but tend to become less so. But many other saṃskāra-s are laid down involuntarily, and some come from past lives.

The great Sanskrit scholar Max Müller, when he was a child, saw a picture of the Brahmins of India and was overwhelmed with a feeling of familiarity; he felt that his destiny lay with India. In fact, this remarkable genius was one of the greatest influences in introducing Far Eastern culture and especially philosophy to the West. His translation of the Upaniṣad-s is still one of the best.

When the saṃskāra-s form a group, reinforcing each other (what we should now call a complex) they are often justified by reasons thought up for the purpose. Ultra-nationalists are an example. Revolutionaries often show the same thing; they can argue clearly against the present regime, but they can give no reason to show that they themselves would do any better. They are against tyranny, but so were Mussolini, Hitler, Stalin, Mao and many other dictators, as can be seen from their early speeches. But they were motivated, perhaps only half-consciously, by saṃskāra-s of envy and love of power.

The yoga psychology shows that everyone worships. We feel that there is something above ourselves, which has absolute value, and we worship it. Some worship money, which for them has a greater value even than life. Periodically misers are found dead in a little room in the big house; they have died of cold because they would have only one bar of the electric fire on. Or they have starved because they would not spend money on food.

Even the most militant sceptics worship something. Djilas, a former Vice-President of Yugoslavia under Tito, who knew Stalin well, said that Stalin, though a materialist, was nevertheless a mystic; in spite of his rejection of some Hegelian doctrine, he worshipped the incarnation of Power, in himself.

The accompanying emotion may be fear. Bertrand Russell, fanatically opposed to religion, admitted (*Dear Bertrand Russell*, Allen & Unwin, 1969) that all his life, at times of deep emotion, he had been terrifyingly overwhelmed by what he himself called 'a Satanic mysticism'. He believed that Joseph Conrad was familiar with the experience and this attracted him strongly to the author of *Heart of Darkness*.

For a view from the sidelines, there is the book by Kazuteru Hitaka (*Ningen Baatorando Rasseru* – The Man Bertrand Russell, 1970, Kodansha, Tokyo). Professor Hitaka, a well-known figure in Japanese intellectual circles and President of the Bertrand Russell Society of Japan, translated a number of Russell's writings, and worked with him for various causes (noting the dislike of Japan as of the USA). He says that Russell loved humanity and was, in the Chinese phrase, 'a seeker of the Way for men to live'. But he was furiously prejudiced against religion (especially in a robe). His jibes at the religious faith of Socrates and Galileo are instances. He had had some semi-mystical experiences, but later was haunted by a sort of demon of doom, more real to him than a bad dream. He tried to meet the attacks with courage, but Hitaka cites a number of passages showing how it could cast him into deepest depression and despair.

Dr Shastri admired some of Russell's earlier work, but said that some of his later writings were from the standpoint of darkness.

'The worship influenced by darkness (tamas)', says the Gītā, 'is of elemental spirits and terrifying forms.' The Hitlers and Himmlers worship astrology and ill-defined racial superstitions. With his almost maniacal faith Hitler was able to capture completely the sceptical mind of Dr Goebbels, his brilliantly successful Minister of Information.

Yoga warns that there is a great danger, even for a good man, in worshipping the divine at large, so to speak. It can lead to a projection of divinity on to something little known, which hardens into fanaticism. The former Dean of Canterbury, Dr Hewlett Johnson, in a number of influential books and writings, exposed his desperate worship of what he called 'the Christian spirit', first in the Soviet Union and then in Mao's China. He was one of the few Westerners to have a personal interview with both Stalin and Mao. He was overwhelmed with what he saw as their spirituality.

With Mao, what struck him most was 'something no picture had ever caught, an inexpressible look of kindness and sympathy, an obvious preoccupation with the needs of others; other people's difficulties, other people's troubles, other people's struggles – these formed the deep content of his thoughts and needed but a touch or a word to bring this unique look of sympathy to his face.' This, he felt, was the true spirit of Christianity which formal Christians so often lamentably failed to practise.

After his interview with Stalin, Hewlett Johnson wrote: 'Stalin is calm, composed, simple, not lacking in humour, direct in speech... nothing cruel or dramatic ... but steady purpose and a kindly geniality.'

Even George Bernard Shaw, so sceptical and iconoclastic in other things, was taken in by Stalin. He had his own mystical vision of a Life Force determined to evolve perfection; but he had no traditionally tested forms in which to worship, so he projected his ideals onto Stalin's Russia.

Such worshippers, some of them very sincere, were in the end worshipping forms created by their own minds. These forms had their power from illusion. What then does the Gītā tell us about worship? What guarantee do we have that traditional forms, like Christ and Kṛṣṇa are anything more than products of mass suggestibility?

One evidence is that texts like the Gītā present us with graded practical experiments. Do these, it says, and you can have direct experience of a God who is not simply your own idea. The experience is no illusion, because it is fruitful in life; it gives not only calm inner clarity, but also inspiration and energy for action. You will come to know the divine purpose in outline, and your own proper part in it in detail.

The second thing is, that the classical forms point beyond themselves. This does not mean that they are untrue. But the Lord reveals these aspects to lead us to higher ones. The traditional forms, assumed by the Lord as an actor puts on clothes, have a lasting charm, a magic about them which attracts the mind and calms the heart. More than that – out of repeated reading of texts and meditations on the form, new things appear.

Much of yoga training is concerned with getting free of domination by saṃskāra-s which constrict the human being to identity with body, family, nation or movement, exclusively, and with hatred of others.

As Dr Shastri says, man can control and change the tendency called Faith; it is not unalterable fate. This is in opposition to a common view today that we are slaves of our 'conditioning'. There is indeed conditioning, but it is not unchangeable. As a matter of fact, experience shows that many teenagers deliberately rebel against their so-called 'conditioning'.

To understand the method of control it is a help to look at a simple example. We must understand the difference between mere repetition and practice. If we look at driving a car, we see that at the beginning, there has to be conscious effort to get some skill. After that the drivers simply repeat, and the process becomes semi-automatic. But they do not improve. Experts say that many drivers never learn the width of their own car, so when overtaking they drive as near the oncoming stream of traffic as they can. This can go on for forty or fifty years. Repetition there is, but not practice. Practice would mean taking the car out and actually learning the width of the car by experiment, perhaps with pegs on an open piece of ground. Mere repetition will not improve the fundamentally defective method of driving; in fact, it reinforces it, although the driver may get more used to handling the car in this wrong way.

Similarly, a two-finger typist does not gradually, 'naturally' as the saying goes, get on to using more fingers. By repetition, he or she gets more skilful at using the two fingers. After ten years or so, some two-finger typists are so familiar with the distances that they can copy-type without looking at the keyboard at all. They have become more skilled at the method, but the method is still a wrong one. Some computer operators today do not learn touch-typing, and it is clear that they never will.

Practice means repeating a process with an ideal before one. When this is done, the execution improves towards the ideal. The improvement is not steady, but in waves.

Chapter XVII Worship, Gift, Austerity

The main part of this chapter, and a good bit of the next (XVIII.18–45) are centred on the effects of the guṇa-s. What the Gītā calls man's 'self nature' (sva-bhāva) consists of tendencies he is born with, as an effect of the saṃskāra dynamic latent impressions laid down in previous births. A selection of some of them, which can consistently manifest together, come together as a block, so to say, determining the conditions of the present birth. It is not unalterable fate, but comparable to the physical make-up of the present body, which can be greatly modified by persistent effort, and by other means also.

The state of the innate nature is reflected in what is technically called one's Faith. This is what one really believes in, as distinct from surface attitudes. The super-nationalist's belief in the divine mission of his group, for which he is willing to die, has often no rational or historical foundation: its basis may be only semi-conscious. Karl Marx did not explain how the Revolution would so change man's nature that he would not simply rebuild an exploitative system again; he just assumed it.

The Gītā gives a three-fold classification of Faith, exemplifying the classes by the beliefs of 'natural' man. Sattvic faith is worship of gods who control the forces of nature and maintain order; rajasic is worship of deities of arbitrary power; tamasic is worship in fear of dark forces felt to be potentially hostile.

There is a strong warning against terrifying self-tortures, chosen and adopted for show or to impress. The Gītā adds that they may be powered by energy of sex desire – in other words, perversions. They impair the body, and impede manifestation of the divine Self in it.

After this warning, the Gītā gives some typical examples of the guṇa-s in various fields of human life. The purpose is to become aware of them in one's conduct, and then change from tamasic and rajasic to the sattvic. In general, the latter are controlled and life-enhancing; the rajasic lead to pain, and the tamasic to delusion.

The chart given below summarizes the main points. Reading across, the same thing – for instance, giving – is shown as dominated by sattva, then by rajas, then by tamas. Reading down the column of a particular guṇa, one can see a picture of someone dominated by it. A common feature of sattvic mind is that it is independent of personal motives and claims on the results of an action; that the action is done; and it is done in serenity.

> XVII.11 Worship done by those not desiring fruit, in a traditional way,
> Thinking simply 'Worship should be performed', with Śamādhi concentration – that worship is of sattva.

17 Austerity performed with highest faith, and not seeking fruits, in concentration of mind –
That austerity is said to be of sattva.

20 The gift to one who makes no return, with the mere thought 'This should be given',
At an appropriate place and time, and to a worthy recipient – That gift is said to be of sattva.

XVIII.26 Free from attachment, not talking of himself, full of firmness and energy,
Unchanged in success or failure – such an agent is called one of sattva.

33 The firmness with which one holds fast the movements of mind, life-currents, and senses,
Unwavering in samādhi – that firmness is of sattva.

The picture of sattvic conduct is sometimes criticized on the ground that it is cold. Simply 'I should give this', and no spontaneous rush of sympathy and compassion. The point will come again: here it can just be said that a rush of emotion, even of kindness, easily arouses other emotions also. A subtle and profound Buddhist analysis remarks that just to seek to do good, without purification of the depths of the mind, can often end up as domination. The fact of helping others means that the helper is in a position of superiority, which can become an unconscious motive, revealing itself as hostility to those not of the same mind. Buddhism has not inspired holy wars or heretic- burning. The sixteenth-century persecution of Christians in Japan was purely political and Buddhist priests took little part in it; the rulers heard that the Spaniards had conquered the Philippines by first creating many Christians to form a fifth column for the subsequent invasion. Christianity has often slipped from St Mark's 'He who is not against us is with us', to St Matthew's 'He who is not with us is against us.'

objects of worship	Sattva	Rajas	Tamas
god	deities of light	deities of power and pleasure	terrifying deities (e.g. the Seven Mothers - Śaṅkara)
food	invigorating, solid, juicy	over-spiced, over-stimulating, ultimately unhealthy	stale, impure
three-fold tapas	concentrated, with faith, desiring no fruit	ostentatious, hypocritical, unstable	deluded, self-torturing, or to gratify spite
sacrifice	not for gain, in proper form, concentrated: 'this should be sacrificed'	to get some fruit, or from mere hypocritical ostentation	contemptuously, casually, sceptically
gift	not for a return, respectfully, to the worthy; 'this should be given'	for some return or gain; or grudgingly	carelessly, contemptuously
renunciation of action	no attachment to action itself, or to any fruits; as duty; 'it is to be done'	giving up duty as too troublesome; futile renunciation	ignorantly and improperly giving up duties
knowledge XVIII.29	*sees* one immortal, undivided in the divided	*sees* various beings of different kinds	*sees* one effect as all; silly; without any real object
action	traditionally prescribed; done without attachment to action or to results; done without love or hate	seeking pleasure, or egoistic; forced through with tiring effort	deluded, inconsiderate, ill-considered

agent	detached, non-egoistic, firm, vigorous, unaffected in success or failure	passionate, greedy, cruel, impure; either elated or depressed	unrealiable, vulgar, unteachable, sly, wicked, lazy, despondent
buddhi (higher mind)	*knows* when to act, and what to do; knows about fear and no-fear, bondage and freedom	*misjudges* right and wrong, what to do and what not to do	*sees* wrong as right, and everything upside down; wholly dark
firmness XVIII.33	controls mind, life-currents and senses by yoga samādhi	successively pursuing virtue, pleasure, ambition, to get their expected results	stupid clinging to sleep, fear, grief, depression, lust
happiness XVIII.37	like poison at first, in the end like nectar, produced by purity of mind in meditation, or vision of Self	like nectar at first, poison in the end taking toll of vigour, wisdom, and success	always self-deluded, based on sleep, indolence, silliness

The Gītā compassion is to see the Self in others, and help towards its realization. Only for this is a gift made and help given, and it must be without any thought of return, and with a serene mind.

Austerity (tapas) is defined in this chapter very widely: it is almost a moral code in itself. There is austerity of the body, austerity of speech, and austerity of the mind.

> XVII.14 Respect to the gods, spiritual men, elders, and the learned,
> Purity, uprightness, control of the instincts, and harmlessness-
> This is called austerity of the body.
>
> 15 Speech that does not provoke, that is true and pleasant and beneficial;
> Also recitation of the holy texts in study
> This is called austerity of speech.

> 16 Inner serenity, kindliness, silence, self-control, and purification of the depths of being –
> This is called austerity of mind.

It is notable again how the Gītā morality stresses the example of the individual life. It believes that the vast majority of the evils besetting humankind are caused not by natural calamities like earthquakes, famine or plague, but by uncontrolled human passions like greed and war, whether national or domestic. The 'silence' referred to in verse 16 refers to the ability to silence the mind in meditation, and to be silent in the face of disaster or provocation.

The three main pillars of Gītā conduct are worship, gift and austerity, each practised without clutching after results of some kind. Some people believe that they do not worship, but in fact the instinct to worship is often repressed, and then projected in unsuitable forms.

Djilas, vice-president of Yugoslavia, who knew Stalin, said: 'Stalin knows everything and can do everything. There is no problem Stalin cannot solve.' After his disillusionment, an interviewer reminded him of these words, which could properly be applied only to God. Djilas said: 'Yes, I think at that time I did worship Stalin.' And he added that his impression was that Stalin mystically worshipped power, and (as mentioned above) himself as a sort of incarnation of power.

The Gītā warns against slipping into such worship, which is of tamas or rajas. Worldly cleverness or strength of will is no defence against perversions of worship. But if the whole personality is tranquillized, purified and steadied, they are seen for what they are.

Chapter XVIII Conclusion

Like Chapter II, this is said by some commentators to be a summary of the teachings of the Gītā. It begins by recalling the familiar distinction between (1) physically giving up (saṃnyāsa) actions, except for a few semi-automatic ones which preserve the body, and (2) energetically performing the actions proper to one's role in life, but without any attachment to the action or to its fruits: this is called tyāga.

The Lord selects worship, gift and austerity as the best of all actions, to typify righteous action in general.

> XVIII.5 Actions of worship, gift, and austerity must not be abandoned, but rather performed;
> Worship, gift, and austerity are purifiers of the wise.
>
> 6 But these actions must be done giving up attachment to them, and all claim on the fruits:
> This is My definite and final judgement.

Then he repeats the point already made several times in the Gītā, that while one has the definite feeling 'I am this body', it is impossible to cease from action. The body would simply perish quite quickly.

> XVIII.11 For a body-wearer cannot give up actions altogether;
> But he who abandons the fruit of action is said to be the man of abandonment.

So far this is the karma-yoga training: proper action is to be done, without attachment, and without claim on fruits in the sense of elation at success or despondency at failure. The action is done by one who feels 'I am this body-mind complex, the agent in this action.' He is technically called a body-wearer, and a mere theoretical knowledge of the truth of the great Self does not change his immediate direct conviction of being the body

We can note that in the listing of the factors of action, the fifth one is the divine will. The first four are: the material basis, the agent, the various instruments, the various activities of the agent. The fifth one, the divine will, does not rule out the power of choice that has been given to the body-wearer human agent: it is to remind him that he alone cannot bring about any effect.

> XVIII.16 He who thinks that it is simply the Self which is the agent of actions,
> Is confused in mind, and fails to see.

Almost immediately, the Gītā presents the truth:

> 17 He whose being is not made-into-an-ego, whose intelligence is not tainted,
> He, even though he slays these people, does not slay, and is not bound.

The body-mind called 'he' slays the people if it is the divine will and inspiration, but the true 'he' is the infinite Self, which neither slays as Arjuna's body is urged to do, nor causes to slay, as the Lord's body as Kṛṣṇa is doing. The great Self is also the true Self of those who seem to be slain. This complements the teaching in II.21, where slaying the Self is shown to be impossible because it is immortal.

In verses 19–30, further vivid illustrations of the influence of the three guṇa-s are given. These have been included in the chart on page 155.

Verses 42–45 give the proper roles of the four classes, who are born with tendencies towards the roles, and must develop and perfect them. Nothing is said in the Gītā about being in a class because born of parents of that class. There is also nothing about privileges. In the Lawbook of Manu, a Brahmin has the privilege of personal immunity from execution even if he has committed murder. The king is directed simply to expel him from the kingdom. The Gītā does not mention anything like this. It speaks not of privileges but rather of duties, such as the Brahmin's duty to speak out the truth; this he must do fearlessly even at risk of his own life.

Some of the points are discussed in the chapter on the Four Vocations (p. 268).

> XVIII.42 Calm, self-control, austerity, purity, patience, uprightness,

Theoretical knowledge and practical realization, faith -
Are the innate impulse-tendencies of Brahmins.

43 Heroism, majesty, firmness, skill, never running away,
Generosity, authority, are innate in Kṣatriya warriors.

44 Skill in agriculture, rearing cattle, trade, are innate to Vaiśya-s;
Action of service is natural to a Śūdra.

Śūdra-s were not helots or slaves. Megasthenes, Greek ambassador in 300 BC, does not mention slaves in his account of Indian society of the time. Some śūdra-s became wealthy, and as Manu notes in passing, even kings. For present-day times, the word 'service' can be taken in its sense of a livelihood or profession whose main aim is to benefit others: public service, welfare service, social service, and so on.

That these classes were seen by the Gītā to be a matter of innate disposition, and not a perhaps uncongenial hereditary role, is shown by the next verse:

45 Taking delight in his own special role, one attains perfection;
Hear now how, delighting in his special action, he attains that spiritual success.

The verse shows that the role is one in which one can delight: it is not a duty done under compulsion against the grain

46 Worshipping with his special action the Lord from whom comes all activity,
By whom all this is pervaded, one attains perfection.

47 Better one's own role, though done imperfectly, than another's part even though well played:
If he does the action proper to his own disposition, he incurs no guilt.

48 The action innate in him should not be given up though it may have some defects:
For all undertakings are clouded by some faults, as fire by smoke.

In connection with performance of the proper role, the Gītā repeats the special words for joy: 'rata' or 'abhi-rata'. They mean 'delighting in', with a sense of complete ease and contentment, and also a nuance of sport. The same word is used of the illumined man engaged in steadying his knowledge: in V.25 and XII.4 he is described as 'delighting in the welfare of all beings.' This is not a duty to be conscientiously carried out, but delight in playing the divine role undiluted by personal considerations.

Then follow a few verses on what follows naturally for this man who has achieved 'perfection' in the form of purity of mind, and transcended action of the form 'I do it'. By solitary meditation, he comes to be settled in his true Self as the attributeless Brahman. The verses summarize teachings on practice in Chapter VI:

> 51 With his mind purified and set in yoga, with firm self-control, Rejecting sounds and other sense-impressions, and putting away love and hate,
>
> 52 In solitude, eating little, restraining speech, body, and mind,
> Always keeping in view his purpose of yoga and meditation, relying on inner independence,
>
> 53 Freed from I-ness, violence, pride, desire, anger and possessiveness,
> Unselfish, serene – he is qualified to become Brahman.

Then the Gītā gives one of its frequent reminders that the supreme Brahman, as the Lord, also projects the world-illusion:

> 54 Having become Brahman, of serene self, he neither grieves nor longs,
> The same to all beings, he attains supreme devotion to Me.

The word para-bhakti, translated as 'supreme devotion', is read by Śaṅkara as awareness of identity with the Lord. It is made clear and undisturbed by the path of jñāna-niṣṭhā, which is in fact a one-pointed current of thought of identity of Self and God. In the end the interior current burns itself away as a mental activity. Patients who have recovered health by a planned regimen under expert guidance, sometimes think, 'I feel really well now, I am healthy.' But after a short time this conception drops away; they enjoy health on a deep level, without thinking about it.

55 By that devotion he comes to know Me, who and what I am in very truth;
Then knowing me in very truth, he enters into Me straightaway.

This verse shows that Knowledge is the cause of instant liberation. But Śaṅkara in his commentary here explains at length that this has to be pure clear Knowledge, mature and without any obstructions. He describes the process: (1) it is truth declared by the holy texts, and (2) presented by the teacher to a pupil (3), who is practised in the twenty qualities listed in XIII.7–11, beginning with Humility and ending with Constancy in Self-knowledge and Perception of the Goal of Knowledge of Truth; (4) it is the truth which has first risen and then matured, which now (5) attains consummation in an absolutely unobstructed experience, immediate identity of Self with the Lord.

The maturing or ripening, mentioned twice in the passage, refers to the path of jñāna-niṣṭhā, clearing away from the uprisen Knowledge any trailing clouds of illusory association. Thus the final stages of the path of Knowledge are summed up.

The Gītā, however, is given formally to a man (and through him to all such men) who has still an individual role in the world. So in the concluding verses it returns to karma-yoga. Karma-yogin-s have not yet realized identity with the Lord in practice.

57 Mentally casting all actions upon Me, devoted to Me,
Keep your mind ever fixed on me by means of yoga.

58 If your mind is on Me, by My grace you will get over all difficulties.
But if from self-will you will not heed, you will perish.

59 Even if from that self-will you resolve not to fight,
Vain would be that resolve: your inner make-up will make you fight.

60 Held fast by your own natural impulse,
What through delusion you tried not to do, you would be driven to do, though unwilling.

These verses can be bewildering at first sight. If Arjuna is going to fight anyway, why the instruction and persuasion to fight? The Lord seems to say that it is not needed. He is predicting that Arjuna, even as he tried to go from the battlefield, would see the arrows begin to fall. He would see his brother Yudhiṣṭhira wounded. In any case his whole warrior training would rise up in explosive fury, and he would rush back to fight.

There is a difference, however. It is the difference between fighting in explosive fury, and fighting as a yogin. As a yogin he will not be driven by passions of rage and hate. He will not fight as the others fight, but will have at least some interior calm, without hatred of those he fights. (He will be all the more effective for that.) It will be done as divine inspiration, and he will be free from fear of death, or failure.

61 The Lord abides in the heart of all beings,
Making them turn about like puppets on a machine, by His magic māyā.

62 Go to Him alone for refuge, with your whole being;
By His grace you will attain supreme peace and the state of immortality.

Verses 61 and 62 give the main teachings in a nutshell: the Lord himself enters all beings, and makes them turn about, controlled as if mechanically by his magic trick-of-illusion called māyā. The Lord himself has entered, as well as constructed, the machine, as Chapter XV explained. He has allowed himself to be deluded. When the deluded Lord turns to the undeluded Lord, his own real Self, with his whole being, the illusion is no longer a bondage; if it is a restriction, that is a voluntary self-restriction.

The verses show that the world-process is willed and purposeful, and that its solution is joy. Dr Shastri compared it to the sport of a very strong swimmer, who deliberately throws himself into a torrent, knowing that he will lose control for a time, but will be able gradually to re-establish it.

The Gītā ends with a verse in which Arjuna's illusion is gone, and he says: 'I will follow your word, and fight.' Śaṅkara explains that he has attained full Knowledge, and has nothing to do as an individual, since he is no longer an individual. The body and mind act without the egoism 'I do': the one Lord shines in his unbroken glory.

It may be asked, what about all the misery seen in the world? The answer of the Gītā is that in those who are drawn to yoga, the Lord is stirring. Most of the misery can be easily alleviated if hearts become free from passion and inertia. Those who are relatively prosperous and secure can contribute materially, but unless hearts are changed, the situation will soon revert to what it was. By practising yoga and purifying their own lives, the partially awakening Lords can help rescue those still spiritually asleep.

Those who complain of the misery and injustice of the world must press the point further. A man asked a spiritual teacher:

'Why does a just God, or a compassionate Buddha, or any of those others they talk about, allow all the evil in the world?'

The teacher replied: 'And do you yourself contribute to this evil which so distresses you?'

Somewhat taken aback, the inquirer thought a bit, and then said in a low voice: 'I am ashamed to say it, but I'd have to admit that I have done things in my life which were unnecessarily cruel, and spiteful too, I suppose. I needn't have done them, but, yes, I did them.'

'Well,' said the teacher, 'You are God, you are Buddha, you are all those others they talk about. Why do you allow yourself to do these things?'

Part III

Śaṅkara on Gītā Practice

The Two Paths

When Arjuna appeals for help, he is not asking for a knowledge of the Universal Self, nor for freedom from the limitations of the world. He wants to know what to do: he is caught in a dilemma, each branch of which is disaster and misery for him and for his world.

In most of the Upaniṣads, on the other hand, the inquirer is one who seeks to know the truth about the universe, or the truth about himself.

> The wife Maitreyi who liked to talk about Brahman (no prejudice against women in the Upaniṣadic tradition) rejects offers of property and says: 'What should I do with that which will not make me immortal? Tell me that which you know, which gives immortality'. (Bṛhadāraṇyaka Upaniṣad)

> Nachiketas refuses similar offers of distraction: 'These things last but till tomorrow. Tell me the secret of death – this is the only boon Nachiketas asks' (Kaṭha Upaniṣad)

These are calm, determined people, who have turned their back on very favourable opportunities, and are bent on knowing the answer to the riddle of the universe and themselves. Some of them have given long service to the teacher, or have proved the strength of their desire to know by terrifying austerities, such as confronting death face to face.

Arjuna's situation is quite different. He is in an emotional crisis, and can see no possible outcome where he could be happy. He is not detached from the world, only crushed by this bit of it. He has not done service to the teacher, only appealed to him impulsively. But there is one point of resemblance: he is desperate. He is willing to do anything, as they are willing to do anything. For this reason the first chapter of the Gītā is called the Yoga of Despair. It differs from mere despair, which is paralysing, because Arjuna appeals to Kṛṣṇa for help. Hope has not been entirely lost. Despair can be turned into a yoga or means when it becomes desperation. As such, the teacher Kṛṣṇa takes advantage of it.

As has been said, he first reminds Arjuna of worldly considerations like his honour as a warrior: this has no effect now. Arjuna has been quoting the words of sages who speak of the disastrous effects of fighting, and the greatness of absolute pacifism.

Kṛṣṇa then speaks of reincarnation.

> II.12 Never did I not exist,
> Nor you, nor these great ones,
> Nor shall we ever cease to be,
> Any of us, in the future.
>
> 13 As in this life, all beings
> Pass through childhood, youth, and age;

In the same way, they pass to another body.
The wise are not confused by such changes.

And again:

II.22 As the wearer casts off worn-out clothes
And puts on himself others which are new,
Even so casting off worn-out bodies,
The body-wearer passes on to new ones.

But Arjuna's distress is too pressing for distant perspectives to relieve it. Kṛṣṇa advises him that his path should be one of action rather than renunciation.

Śaṅkara's Presentation of the Gītā Paths

Yoga means a method, and in the Gītā several times the Lord teaches two methods: the method of Action (karma-yoga), and the method of Knowledge (jñāna-yoga). Note that Knowledge too is a method, which is often called Renunciation, because that is its chief characteristic.

In a few places, the Lord says that the Action path is better than, or easier than, the Knowledge path of renunciation. From these statements, it can be supposed that the paths are self-contained alternatives. It is tacitly assumed that the path of Action is for an extravert who feels alive only when acting. The path of Knowledge is then thought to be for an intellectual introvert who acts only reluctantly. In spite of his actual experience that he is the body, this withdrawn introvert is supposed to cherish a belief, or hope, that somehow he is not. The Gītā is then cited to the effect that either path, followed through to the end, will give liberation. That is supposed to be either a state of active and interested divinity (for the extravert, who somehow always keeps his characteristics even in transcendence) or a state of featureless abstraction (for the introvert).

But Śaṅkara holds the Upaniṣadic view that the path of Action comes *first*, to be *followed* by the path of Knowledge. The Gītā itself says (V.6) that Knowledge-renunciation can hardly be attained without having performed Action yoga. This modifies the previous statement that one alone might be enough. Śaṅkara has the first discussion of the Two Paths in II.21. He quotes the revered Vyāsa, reputed author of the Mahābhārata epic itself: 'There are two paths.... Of these, the path of Action comes first, then the path of Knowledge.'

The analysis has already been looked at. It can be summed up:

The State of Ignorance

'I do this to get that result for myself. I am happy or sad. I age and die.'

Yoga of Action (karma-yoga)

'I do this, but whatever the result I remain calm, through meditation practice (III.7). I submit my feelings to God and meditate on him.'

Yoga of Knowledge-Renunciation (jñāna-yoga)

'I do not act at all, though body and mind may continue to act. The freedom of the great Self casts off false memories of bondage.'

The clue to Śaṅkara's arguments against opponents is that the opponent takes renunciation in the literal sense of living as a beggar-monk. The Gītā says that in itself this has no value. Śaṅkara shows that the Gītā teaches two inner renunciations: (a) renouncing the fruits of action, and later on, all self-interested actions; this is karma-yoga renunciation; (b) renouncing the whole feeling 'I do', out of realization of the great Self. The central feature of both paths is meditation, practised in stillness but finally interpenetrating the whole of life.

There is a parallel with mastering a foreign language. To be a master, one must be able to speak and hear, read and write, freely and with individual expression. He must be able to do this even when angry or depressed. He must also be able to understand and express (not necessarily agree with) the foreign thoughts and concepts for which his own language has no words.

He has to begin with grammatical structures, preferably under a teacher. To try to learn 'naturally, from the people' leads, for example, to pidgin English – comprehensible, but confined to elementary levels.

As he gets skill, he can translate internally foreign sentences he hears, and translate some of his own thoughts into correct foreign sentences. But that language is still something other, from which and into which he translates.

In yoga, this corresponds to karma-yoga – he translates his natural feelings and impulses into spiritual ones; he worships God, but as something other.

In the language study, the time comes when some of the foreign words occasionally appear spontaneously in response to a situation. Now is the time when he has to make a jump. He has to trust himself to think in that language, and allow the thought to express itself directly. It takes some courage to do this, and some experts fail to make the leap. Their use of the language then always remains awkward and often pedantic. But for those who make the leap (and usually it has to be made a number of times) the foreign language is now part of himself. There is no otherness about it. Still, it can take a little time before old habits of 'inner translation' drop away, and it is firmly established.

In the yoga, the time comes when the essence is purified, and shafts of light from the divine occasionally appear. Then the jump has to be made from worship of a divine other into being the divine Self. This too takes courage, and some draw back. But, as the Gītā says, finally the Lord manifests himself in the heart, and limitations fall away.

Even then it can take a little time before memories of individual agency are dropped off completely, and the discarding process is what is meant by Knowledge-yoga.

Śaṅkara presents the stages of the two paths again and again. Typical is the commentary on V.12:

Karma-yoga

the steady-minded one (yukta = set in samādhi-meditation).
'I do actions for the Lord alone' – giving up personal claim to the fruits
purity of mind (sattva-śuddhi)

Knowledge-yoga

attainment of Knowledge ('I am That')
abandoning action (physically, or by thought – V.13)
Knowledge-devotion (jñāna-niṣṭhā – casting off delusive memories)

Freedom

Mokṣa – transcendental peace

Śaṅkara makes the point that the karma-yogin cannot practise the Knowledge path, because he still feels 'I am acting'. While that is his living experience, his repetition of a Knowledge text like 'I am the unchanging Self' will have no conviction at all. However Dr Shastri told pupils practising devotion to the Lord as external, that the time would come in the meditation when the Lord would reveal a glimpse of himself within. At that time their practice would become Knowledge. Then on returning to the world, they could practise devotion again on the karma-yoga basis.

Illusion

Why is it that the Gītā so often puts the texts of the two paths close together? It is because ordinary experience is based on a sort of illusion.

Some of the classical examples of this kind of illusion are outside our normal experience, and make no impact on a Western reader. In India, to 'see' a snake where there is only a rope can give quite a little shock, and to an Indian the example is telling.

But many Western people have never seen a snake outside the Zoo. As Indians say humorously: 'If you saw a snake, you would call the police!' Since, then, we never see snakes, we do not see illusory snakes either.

I realized this when with a friend I was looking for something in a London flat. I whisked open the door of a big wall cupboard. It happened that a thick black belt, kept on the top shelf, had fallen down, and one end of it must have got caught on the little bolt inside the cupboard door. The effect was, that when I quickly pulled open the door, this black sinuous length came shooting out on to the floor. Having had a couple of snake experiences in a house in India, I reacted quickly. My eyes told me: 'Snake!' I saw a snake, and jumped back. But my companion stood there calmly as the belt came to rest by his feet; he told me afterwards that he wondered what it was, but it never occurred to him that it was alive. He saw no snake.

Śaṅkara analyses such a case of illusion: it is the appearance, as a living sense-experience, of a memory of a real snake seen previously somewhere else, and now projected on to something similar. A common form of this illusion in India used to be that a man is walking along in the dusk, swinging a lantern: he sees a snake lying on the ground to one side. It is moving a little: he knows it is a snake. He has a fright and cautiously retreats (cautiously because snakes often move about in pairs). Then a friend sees him and calls out: 'It's all right; that's a rope. It just dropped off the cart and I was coming back for it.' He carefully goes near, and finds it is indeed a rope. Its apparent movement had been a reflection of his own movement; the shadow of the rope was moving because it was cast by his own moving lantern.

The illusion, though unreal, has effect. Śaṅkara remarks in his great commentary on the Brahma Sūtra-s that sometimes an imaginary poison can kill a man. A doctor in Malaya described in his memoirs how he was called out to a plantation to treat a snake-bite. A planter had come back home, rather drunk, and flung himself fully dressed on to his bed. He felt a convulsion beneath him, jumped up in a panic, and found that the crash of his body had killed a snake which had crept in between the sheets. It was still moving in the death convulsions. In the confusion, the planter had scratched his arm on a splinter of the wooden bed frame, but he got the idea that the snake had bitten him before it died. By the time the doctor arrived, the cut seemed to be inflamed, and the man was sweating with pain. The doctor saw at once that this was no snake-bite, but knew that his patient was in no condition to listen – the pain was proof enough that the snake had injected some poison. The doctor wrote in the memoir that he knew from experience that such a belief could cause very serious symptoms. He therefore immediately treated the injury as a snake-bite, and remarked after a minute: 'You're lucky: he only just got in a scratch. He'd no time to chew on it and give you a real shot. What's there is dispersing already; the alcohol doesn't help, of course, but you're throwing it off. ...' He chattered away, and after a few minutes the pain began to disappear. Much later, he told him what had really happened to him. The doctor did not argue with the patient's fixed idea; he treated him according to his conviction. When the sufferer is no longer in a state of agitation, he will be able to listen, and understand the truth.

The victim is not always to be saved. Dr Shastri told his pupils of a case in India which he saw as a boy. A house roof was to be rethatched. As the old thatch was being taken off in handfuls one worker – a simple man – found that he had picked up in his handful a dead snake. 'It must have bitten me,' he cried, and began to tremble. It was explained to him that the snake must have been dead for some time, but in spite of all that could be done, he himself was dead in three days.

Many illusions can have such marked physical effects; the examples of 'snake-bite' are not unique. In many cases of illness there is an added element produced by fearful imaginings. An old farmer has related how, when he was a boy, they were still branding young sheep. The first time he was called to help his job was to hold the legs. The sheep gave a piteous cry as it was branded, and after a little he began to feel a pain on his own side, corresponding to where the hot brand was applied to the sheep.

He was soft-hearted, and it got so bad that he could not go on. His uncle the farmer understood, and told him: 'Well, sit down over there. Don't look at us, but look at the sheep that have been done.' He saw to his surprise that the little sheep cried for only about a minute, and then began grazing. After that they once or twice stopped and gave a small cry, but soon seemed to have forgotten all about it. As he watched, he found the pain in his own side disappearing.

An experiment which has been successfully performed many times, though barred today on ethical grounds, is to suggest to a blindfolded volunteer that he is touched by a glowing iron rod. Strong reddening and, in some cases, blisters result. Anatomists have wondered how the sympathetic nerve, the only organ linking the brain and the skin, could evoke a particular local effect like a blister. There is a critical review of the literature reporting controlled experiments on these lines, and the conclusion is that such effects do occur.

The classical illustrations of illusion given so far have been negative. They are unfortunate accidents, which have frightening or dangerous effects. Sometimes Śaṅkara extends the snake-rope illusion, along with its unfavourable effects, to the world-illusion. The world-appearance then becomes something to be avoided, dispersed as soon as possible. This is a viewpoint appropriate for one who has completed his role in life and has retired from the world. Perhaps he has become a monk-teacher.

However, the Gītā gives a different view for people committed by their past undertakings to action in the world. Śaṅkara too cites other kinds of illusion, this time deliberately created for a hidden purpose. A modern example might be a big city in Japan, where police seem to be everywhere. They are standing watchfully at street comers, traffic intersections, and near motorways. A foreigner feels he is under constant surveillance, and is on his best behaviour all the time. One day he happens to pass close to one of the policemen and finds that it is a life- size model. After that he develops a little rule: if it moves, it is a policeman, and if it does not, it is a dummy. Then one day, he parks illegally under the nose of one of the models, having watched it for a minute or so to check that it does not move. It then charges him with his offence. Japanese police are trained to stand quite still for ten-minute spells: the model is made to look like a policeman, and the policeman is trained to look like a model. It is a double false attribution, and this too is a feature of Śaṅkara's philosophy.

There is yet another type, where an illusion is created not only to give significance but also to create beauty. Śaṅkara cites the drama in this connection. It was favoured by Dr Shastri in his exposition of the Gītā. This depends on an illusion cast over the audience by the performance, and partially accepted by them. When the popular theatre was still comparatively new, audiences used to hiss the villain, and sometimes try to warn the hero. In a dim way they still knew that they had paid for their seats. They knew with one part of the mind that what they saw was merely actors playing a part. But the illusion could grip them so strongly that they felt it as real. At performances of *Dracula* there were first-aid staff in attendance to look after those who fainted.

We may feel more sophisticated today, but television stations often receive letters from viewers which show that they think they have been looking at real events. When a popular elderly actress complains (following her script) of migraine headaches, sometimes more than a dozen letters come to her, addressed to the station giving remedies for migraine which the writers have found effective. Research shows that there are many more viewers, who do not actually write, but still have difficulty in distinguishing reality from illusion. In one episode of a popular serial, then running over thirty years, one of the female characters was to retire to the country. The script made the mistake of mentioning an actual village. Some fans of the programme found it on the map, then made the trip and knocked up various houses to ask where they could find her. Apologizing, the programme producer remarked that some regular viewers find difficulty in distinguishing the levels of reality. 'We should have known', he added sadly.

Both types of illusion – accidental and purposeful – are given by the Gītā, and by Śaṅkara following the Gītā. The first type, where the illusion itself has no value, is given when the impact of events in the world seems shattering. In XVIII.61 the Gītā says that most men and events are like mere puppets, with only a semblance of choice, mechanically and mindlessly driven by a magic illusion (māyā). Moreover, even the wise follow their nature; what should forcible restraint avail (III.33)? Again, all beings come into manifestation, and then inevitably go out of manifestation again; it is meaningless to grieve over what is unavoidable (II.28). In one place the Gītā calls the world 'joyless'; it tells the disciple to do his duty and then leave it. These passages are directed to those who feel tightly bound by the world as absolutely real. Just so the parents might say to a child overwhelmed by the reality of a pantomime in which the hero-children seem certain to be killed: 'It's not real. There's nothing there at all. It's just actors coming on and off the stage.'

But there is the other type of illusion, where the wonder and divine beauty of the world are appreciated. It is a spiritual play, put on by the magical power of the Lord and entered into by him. In this, human beings also have a part which they can play. They can have some choice, and can voluntarily and consciously co-operate with the Lord instead of being puppets. This view is for those who feel the stirrings of freedom in themselves. In some of the audience and actors, the Lord begins to awaken to his own display of māyā.

The world-play is accepted as partially real, by the voluntary consent of audience and actors. If the children in the audience at *Treasure Island* believe that the jewels on the stage in the final scene are real, they may want to have them, and even try to climb up on to the stage to get them. But simply to dismiss them as totally valueless in every sense, destroys enjoyment of the play. In *Julius Caesar*; if the actor in the title role thinks that the daggers of the assassins are real, he may fight desperately for his life. If he simply dismisses them as fake stage knives, he will not fall dead. For successful drama, there has to be a balance between belief and disbelief. Some degree of belief is necessary to see the beauty of a masterpiece like *King Lear*: but if belief became absolute, the scene where Gloucester's eyes are put out would scar the viewer for a long time.

There are differences between the world as generally experienced, and a play. These differences are confronted in the life of yoga. Still, the play analogy, though not perfect, teaches one more thing. There is a continuous strain in maintaining an illusion, even unconsciously. Television viewers usually believe that they are in relaxation, but this is not so. It is an effort to keep masking out the inconsistencies, and hold the sense of a living reality in the tiny screen figures, which yet speak with normal full-size voices.

In fact the whole world of television is light and nothing but light, produced in a mysterious way by electrons fired from the back of the set on to the screen. It is mysterious because, the physicists say, the path of each electron is unpredictable. The picture is reasonably sharp only because the number of electrons involved is enormous: by the law of averages, the cumulative effect of many electrons is predictable. But there is no known reason why any particular electron should go to point x rather than some other place. The picture fragment is an event without a cause.

These facts are worth mentioning because there are some parallels with Śaṅkara's analysis of the world as perceived by us. Strictly speaking the universe too is an event without a cause, though a cause is provisionally postulated. But yoga practice does not depend on distant inferences from present-day physics. Yoga is derived from its own experiments directly on consciousness, and not from inferences or guesses.

Interpretation

Śaṅkara established his standpoint by commenting on sacred texts such as Upaniṣad-s and the Gītā. The latter is the Upaniṣad-s put into verse for aspirants heavily involved in worldly concerns. He insists that he is presenting nothing new. He wrote a short commentary on the Chapter of the Self in one of the law-books, and a lengthy one on the Yoga Sūtra-s of Patañjali. He wrote at least one independent work, called the Thousand Teachings. A couple of others, out of the very many attributed to him, may be authentic. But he saw himself primarily as a transmitter of the holy truth which passed through the Upaniṣad-s.

He interprets his texts by putting others alongside them, and applying constructive reasoning. The reasoning is constructive because the texts record actual experience of ancient sages; that experience can be, and must be, confirmed by students of the present day who want to free themselves from suffering. Śaṅkara's interpretations are made on the basis of a tradition of experiment and confirmation.

He knows that words alone cannot describe supra-mental experience accurately. The mind itself can attain no more than a glimpsed reflection of Reality. Nevertheless he believes that words can give practical instruction as to what to seek and how to seek it.

Contradictions

Seemingly contradictory doctrines are given in the Gītā; for instance, the doctrine of the three guṇa-s. Śaṅkara remarks that this is not the highest truth, but says it is useful.

In the same way, a bone could be analysed by a biologist in terms of function, apparently purposeful; by a chemist, as molecular structure, in terms of apparently purposeless determinism; by a physicist, as subatomic particles, undetermined and puzzlingly non-local. The three analyses may not have too much to do with each other. Still it is recognized that they are not necessarily contradictory, but to be distinguished in terms of depth.

Borrowings

Certain similarities of doctrine can be pointed out between Śaṅkara and some Buddhists. It is theorized that the later must therefore have borrowed from the earlier. But this idea rests on an unspoken assumption that the doctrines are in any case mere speculations. The assumption is false.

If in a present-day adventure story... the reader finds a map very similar to that in *Treasure Island*, or *The Lord of the Rings*, it is reasonable to suppose borrowing. But if we look at a nineteenth-century ordnance map of Iceland, and compare it with the similar map of Iceland today, there is no question of borrowing. Both of them were based on surveys of an existent island. They are alike because they are based on the same thing.

In the same way, descriptions of spiritual experiences, and corollaries drawn from them, can be similar because they are based on the same thing.

Interpretation

The commentator on the Gītā fills out the meaning of the verse in three main ways. First, by putting alongside it other verses from the Gītā itself, and from the Upaniṣad-s, and from other authoritative texts of the tradition. But the mere bringing together of texts is not enough. If there is already some pre-conception in the mind of the one who selects the texts, they can be selected to mean something against the whole spirit of a text, however holy.

For instance a hostile critic can bring together texts from the New Testament to show that Christ taught hatred: 'If anyone comes to me, and does not hate his father and mother, wife and children, brothers and sisters, even his own life, he cannot be a disciple of mine' (Luke 14.26); 'You must not think I have come to bring peace to the earth; I have come to bring not peace but a sword. I have come to set a man against his father, a daughter against her mother, a son's wife against her mother-in-law,... and a man will find his enemies under his own roof.' Such texts should not be ignored. They are riddles, set by Christ systematically to give the minds of his hearers a shake to stimulate them to untie the knot.

So the second requirement for interpretation is that the texts should be selected, and treated, by one who knows from experience what they are pointing towards. But this too is not quite enough.

To rule out self-delusion, a teacher's experience must agree with that recorded by the traditional teachers. Everyone who completes the training comes to the same state. In order not to confuse the people, he should present his experience in the traditional forms. Nevertheless there is always something new in it, which attests to living inspiration.

The Indian tradition tried to get precision in words and concepts. Still, they recognized that words have limitations. It would take many words to describe the outline of a tree: one glance could tell one more.

The Pyramids of Gizeh have been well-known as a Wonder of the World for over 4,000 years. A traveller writes: 'The Pyramids were small black triangles against the dawn', and another: 'The Pyramids are the most massive structures yet put together by man.' Because we fill in the unspoken assumptions, we do not find the statements contradictory.

But then we read a guidebook which says: 'Any active person can easily climb the crumbling stones of the Great Pyramid, and the same with the Second Pyramid.' Another guidebook says: 'Anyone reasonably energetic can climb the Great Pyramid, but ropes are needed for the Second Pyramid'. This is a flat contradiction as it stands, but it is resolved by one glance at a picture or drawing. The smooth casing still remains at the top of the Second Pyramid. The seeming contradiction is from the ambiguity of the word 'climb'; to climb a tree does not necessarily mean to the very top.

In the same way, the classical commentator treats the texts in the light of experience, confirmed by generation after generation of teachers. The maps of the holy texts are read and explained by a traveller who has himself passed that way.

In his commentary to the Brahma Sūtra, Śaṅkara explains that Śruti (literally 'hearing') is the sacred text of revelation of truth.

It is the experience of the divine sages, expressed as far as words will allow. But he points out that words can be no more than indications; words and thoughts are not experience-of-truth itself. They are limited by the mind which conceives the expressions, and never more than that.

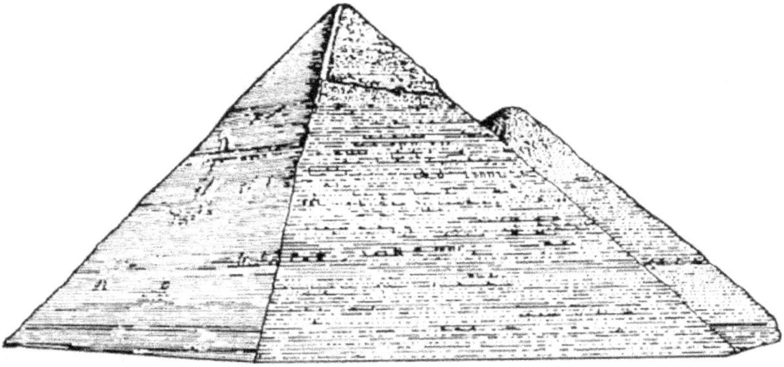

Second Pyramid (*left*), Great Pyramid (*right*)

Just so a map, or a signpost, can never be completely accurate. But if several of them are collated, there is much greater precision. Śaṅkara's method is to bring together holy texts referring to the same truth; the mind comes to complete immobility on it. Then there is a jump as mind is transcended and truth realized directly, not through concepts.

It may be necessary to resolve apparently conflicting and contradictory passages in the texts, and this is done by the commentator. It is not a question of verbal and intellectual ingenuity; the commentator must himself realize the truth being indicated.

Outline of Practice

Independence

Verses on independence of the opposites come in nearly every chapter. The instruction is first about physical effects:

> II.14 It is the contacts with material things that cause heat and cold, pleasure and pain;
> They come and go, impermanent as they are,
> Do you endure them bravely.

Śaṅkara points out that some, such as heat and cold, register on the senses, and these are invariable effects. Other opposites like pleasure and pain are appreciated by mind, and the same thing can have varying mental effects. For instance, a given degree of heat or cold can give pleasure in one situation and pain in another. A nearby blazing fire might be intolerable on the equator, but welcome in the Arctic. Śaṅkara stresses the emotional element involved in pleasure and pain. In one of his other commentaries, he gives the example of a father delightedly lifting his newborn son high above his head; the tiny boy makes a mess all over him. The father does not resent it at all, but laughs happily.

The Gītā says that pains are to be endured bravely, realizing that they will all pass. Pleasures too are impermanent, and if they become urgent impulses, they lead to pain. Manu says that the momentary relief found in gratifying a pleasure-impulse is like trying to put out a fire by throwing liquid butter on it. The flames do indeed die down, but almost immediately they spring up again with redoubled vigour. In yoga, the pleasure/pain alternation is compared to a fever, when the sick body twists and turns to get some relief. There is a momentary pleasure experienced with each new body position, but the relief passes off quickly and the position becomes intolerable. This is not to say that sensible nursing (not indulgence) is a waste of time; it can lessen the discomfort. But there is no peace till the fever is cured. So in the world, though some shifts and manoeuvres can lessen the sufferings of life-in-illusion, there is no peace till its fever has been cured.

The Gītā analysis is that life has an underlying background of suffering, because of the felt restrictions on freedom of the spirit. To that extent it is like a prison camp, set in barren country, as many of them are. Our present attempts to extract pleasure from life-as-it-is are like the entertainments got up by prisoners from time to time: songs, plays, charades, skits and so on. They have almost no material, but somehow they improvise. It is a brave attempt to forget the prison, a conscious return to childhood. For a short time there can be a real delight in preparing and watching these things. They are a splendid defiance of the sufferings of the situation.

But suppose the guards have abandoned the camp during the night, because their own side is retreating. Now there is nothing to stop prisoners from walking out. The guards may have delayed this by putting dummies in the watchtowers, which are still apparently manned. When this is discovered, to put on a camp show would be merely silly. The proper joy would be in preparing for the journey across the semi-desert, to join the friendly forces. That is, yoga.

Another example, given by Śaṅkara, is eating poisoned sweets. One who does not know about the poison eats happily; the pain comes only later. One who knows has a background of suffering all the time, though he too gets the tiny enjoyment from the sweetness. Why would he eat it? We see today how some diabetics cannot resist sweets which they know are poison for them. But if they are clear-minded, they soon correct the tendency to lapse.

A third pair of opposites, more dangerous because more subtle, is honour-and-power and disgrace. Acts of kindness may be powered by a hidden desire to dominate, or to be admired. Such subtle pleasures may be aimed at only semi-consciously, but their influence goes deep. Similarly many people find disgrace and scorn harder to bear than physical pain. A deep physical wound, if washed and protected by a bandage, will generally heal in the end. But wounds left by venomous tongues may never heal, because they are constantly re-opened in memory. Dr Shastri remarked that one of the tests of a really great man is that he can pass through a hail of slander and ridicule without losing his inner balance.

How is independence to be practised? It is recommended to begin with small things: to miss a meal occasionally, going on to fasting one day a month; to sit up once a month for two or three hours in meditation, going on to a whole night of study and meditation. (Gamblers have no difficulty in sitting up all night for their addiction.)

However, if such things are individually chosen, they lose some of their value. Most of us choose only what we feel we shall be good at. Trainers in physical skills know well that it is essential to tackle the weak points; few people will do this on their own, and a teacher is a great help. It should be added that some pupils, when the teacher insists on their practising at the weak points, instead of the strong ones where they can shine, claim that the teacher does not 'understand' them. Later they are grateful to him.

However, for sincere aspirants, the situations of life become teachers. If they are taken as occasions for practice of independence, the development will be complete. When caught in a storm without a raincoat or any shelter, to walk straight ahead, without futile inner complaints, is practice; to try to feel the inner Self independent of the body, is spiritual practice.

It is well known that in a crisis, physical pains are hardly noticed; the same thing can happen also in a calm environment. The Hungarian chess master Maroczy had a fine moustache, of which he was proud. During one tournament game he was resting his chin on his right hand, in an attitude common among chess players. But it was observed that he was slowly pulling out the hairs of the right side of his moustache, one by one, as he considered his moves. It is an exquisitely painful little operation, but he was unconscious of that. No one dared to interrupt. At the end of the game he was amazed to find blood on his face, and half his moustache gone. He now had to shave off the other half. Such incidents, showing the overwhelming importance of the mental element in apparently basic physical experiences, are not too infrequent. It is worth collecting a few from reports in the Press or books, to help cultivate independence.

Again, even severe pain is bearable if it is undergone voluntarily, and for a constructive purpose. A sprinter sometimes collapses in agony at the end of a race; it may take some time to recover. When he does, he immediately wants to race again. If the same pain were forcibly inflicted on him by a third party, it would rightly be called torture.

In one tradition, a yogin who has to face severe pain is recommended to slow down and deepen his breathing for at least ten minutes beforehand. At the actual moment, he is to hold his breath. Where it is feasible, this can take the keen edge off pain.

Śaṅkara adds a new element to the bare practice of courageous independence, as taught in the early chapters of the Gītā. This is, that all experiences and events are to be taken as from the hand of the Lord. It is not a question of praying that the circumstances may be changed, but to take them as they are, as opportunities for spiritual growth. We may take vigorous action to improve unfavourable surroundings, but in so far as they cannot be changed, the hand of the Lord is seen even in difficulties and sufferings. Then the suffering will be reduced, and an underlying joy glimpsed.

One may think: 'If the adverse or frightening things stay as they are, the suffering will stay as it is. Ideas about the Lord will not make any actual difference.' But they will: the situation is transformed. There is an example from one of the traditional knightly arts of Japan.

Up to some fifty years ago, in the art called Judo, to attain First Dan, with the right to wear a Black Belt, was a great event in a pupil's life. (The standard required for First Dan was then higher than today.) Some of the young men who got it could become excited, and the teacher and seniors of their practice hall used to take measures to deflate that first euphoria. When the new Dan came on to the mats, with his brand new belt, the old teacher would call him for a practice. Now there are certain rather rough techniques which were never shown in the early years, and the teacher would use a couple of these to surprise and throw the youngster very heavily. After that practice, before he could even get his breath, he would be called out by a tough senior, again using contest tricks which he had never seen. Then another of the contest team, and yet another. By this time he would be dripping with sweat, totally exhausted, and frightened. These experienced contest experts, so genial before, now were frowning and apparently trying to injure him. Perhaps they don't want another Black Belt, and are trying to get rid of me? They are running wild. All sorts of panicky thoughts. Many who passed through this experience have testified how bewildering and terrifying it could be.

No help from anyone. Then looking despairingly round the hall, he sees the old teacher standing with his arms folded, watching. The discipline in the training hall is absolute. If that teacher clapped his hands once, everyone would stand perfectly still. Suddenly the victim knows, that all this is controlled, watched, and somehow for his own good: it will never go too far. His muscles ache, he is still exhausted, still gasping for breath. But he knows that this is for him, not for them, and he is grateful, and – a long way down – he is content.

Life/death is one of the great pairs of opposites. The yoga does not recommend mere faith in immortality: faith, like any other idea, is liable to change when unsupported. By samādhi meditation and other practices of karma-yoga, the yogin must attain a glimpse of immortality in this very life. Such a direct glimpse will free him from the fear of annihilation. This is the final complete independence of the opposites.

Worship for Sceptics

The steps in yoga, says Patañjali's Yoga Sūtra, are: Faith, Energy, Memory, Samādhi meditation, Prajñā-knowledge, 'That rules me out', replies the sceptic; 'one cannot believe to order. I don't accept these things in the first place.'

'You are not asked to believe', replies yoga, 'it is suggested only that you experiment.'

Yoga makes its own experiments. It investigates consciousness directly, and does not depend on inferences from experiments on material events. It gives methods which can, and must, be tried. Without actual trial, yoga would be no more than a rather unlikely theory. A few things are assumed for a time, as working ideas, but they have to be experienced directly before they are finally taken as true.

One such assumption is that there is an all-powerful, unlimited, creator and controller, who projects himself in limited forms to help seekers to realize him. The forms may be human, such as the traditional forms of Kṛṣṇa, Christ, the Buddhas; or abstract, such as the order and upward progress in nature including human nature.

'Yes, yes, yes', interrupts the critic, 'we have all heard this sort of thing. But where is the direct experimental evidence you promised?'

Yoga continues: 'Here is the setting for one definite experiment. First, the principle. The supreme Spirit is all-pervading, and therefore also present in the depths of the heart and mind of man. While the heart is full of conflicting desires, hopes and fears and so on, the light of the Spirit within is obscured, as the bright sky is obscured by masses of storm clouds. Devotion and meditation directed to one of the divine forms will thin the veils, outer and inner. They become in places like the thin white clouds, and the supreme Spirit begins to be seen in the outer world, and finally within also. The yogin becomes more and more aware of the divine purpose, and the role he can play as part of it.

'Now, the actual practice. It depends on the fact of resonance between the external forms of the Lord, and the Lord seated within the heart, as the texts say. The experimenter is asked to study a traditional text on one of the traditional forms. He should undertake to read it with attention at least 20 minutes every morning, in a quiet place.'

Let us suppose for instance, that the form chosen is Jesus, and the experimenter is reading the Fourth Gospel. If he is attentive, some unusual point in the text will strike him. The holy texts are full of such small riddles, as they seem. He must not pass over them: they are openings.

Take it that he has come to John 7.53: an incident in the Temple. The popular memory of this story is that the young woman was accused before Jesus of an offence punishable by stoning. He invented the inspired answer: 'Let him who is without sin cast the first stone.' And the accusers went away.

But that is only a part of the story. Here it is in the New English Bible translation:

> At daybreak he appeared again in the temple, and all the people gathered round him. He had taken his seat and was engaged in teaching them when the doctors of the law and the Pharisees brought in a woman caught committing adultery. Making her stand in the middle, they said to him, 'Master, this woman was caught in the very act of adultery. In the Law, Moses has laid down that such women are to be stoned. What do you say about it?' They put the question as a test, hoping to frame a charge against him. Jesus bent down and wrote with his finger on the ground. When they continued to press their question, he sat up straight and said, 'That one of you who is faultless shall throw the first stone.' Then once again he bent down and wrote on the ground. When they heard what he said, one by one they went away, the eldest first; and Jesus was left alone with the woman still standing there. Jesus again sat up and said to the woman, 'Where are they? Has no one condemned you?' She answered, 'No one, sir.' Jesus said, 'Nor do I condemn you. You may go, and do not sin again.'

The practice would be to read this passage, visualizing the scene, and memorizing a sentence from the teaching given. One should look for the deeper meaning. Often when a holy text is read, a supposedly pious reader gives up thinking. 'It is all very holy and doubtless means something exalting, but it is not for us to pry.' In yoga however equal attention is focussed on just such things.

With this in mind, let us look at the story. Scholarship can tell us a few extra points, though not the central meaning. It can tell us for instance that Jesus would have been teaching in one of the courtyards of the Temple, quite likely in Solomon's Portico, which is later named in John's Gospel as a place where he taught. It also tells us that at this time of Passover, more than a quarter of a million pilgrims came to the Temple to make offerings. Their feet would have brought in a good deal of sand from the roads, so the ground of such courtyards would have been sandy.

Again it tells us that this woman would have been a newly betrothed girl caught with a man, in violation of her solemn vows. He could make a break for it, but she had nowhere to go. She was brought before Jesus, apparently in the hope of trapping him with an awkward choice: 'The Law of Moses says that such should be killed by stoning.' Such a punishment was not too rare; Jesus himself was later saved from it only by a miracle.

Scholarship also tells us that the sentence: 'That one of you who is faultless shall throw the first stone', was not an invention of Jesus. If it had been, the effect might not have been so immediate. He was in this case, as in some others, skilfully putting together two texts from the Law. The accusers were quoting the Law to support their case, and now that very Law was turned on them. The two texts state, that the witnesses must be 'of good character', and 'one of the witnesses shall throw the first stone'. Both come from Deuteronomy, the same book the accusers were quoting.

However all this does not explain the central point. What is that point?

Jesus, who was sitting, bent forward and wrote with his finger on the ground. This is the only place where the Gospels describe him as writing. Getting no reply, they pressed forward and asked him again. He straightened up, looked at them, and said, 'That one of you who is faultless shall throw the first stone.' Then he bent forward and wrote on the ground again.

These were scholars, and they are described as pressing forward round Jesus, so they would instinctively read what he had written in the sand of the Temple court. After the second writing, our text says only that they went out, the eldest first. The rest of the story is well-known.

Now as an example of the yogic method of thinking about a text as well as just reading it: what did he write? He wrote twice, and after the second writing they went out. What was it in the sand, that made them go out, the eldest first?

And why did he not speak it? He did speak the words about the one without sin. So why did he not speak this too, whatever it was?

The Gospels have a number of such riddles; the sceptic is asked to notice them, and then try to solve them. A keen reader will have a little illumination when he solves one. To do so will produce a resonance from the Jesus in his own heart.

There have been a few attempts to solve this one, some of them trivial. For instance, it has been suggested that he was simply doodling on the ground, to show complete lack of interest in the proceedings. But he was not disinterested, for he spoke the two texts from the Law.

At the risk of weakening the force of inquiry, it may be mentioned that St Jerome proposed a much deeper solution. Even this explains only a part of the riddle. He says that Jesus listed their sins, point by point, on the ground. We know from several incidents in the Gospels that he could look at people and see their inmost heart. But in that case, why write it? Why not look at each one and say. 'You have done this, and you have done that. So you are no true witnesses of good character. You cannot stone another when you are sinners yourselves'?

Why did he write, and why did he write twice, and why did the eldest go out first?

One who reads attentively the life of an avatar will come across such places. When one catches his mind, he should think about it. He should stop reading and think about it. Then he should re-read it slowly, visualize the scene, filling in the details sentence by sentence. He will find it easy to think about it in spare moments during the day. If after a week he has no answer, he goes on with the text, till another incident catches his attention.

After a month, the whole text may be changed. The Rāmāyana, the Bhagavad Gītā, some of the spiritual stories in the Masnavi of Rumi or the collections of Zen stories, are suitable texts for striking a spark.

If he persists, with the same interest that a short-wave radio enthusiast seeks for a distant station, there will be a stir within him. His experiment is beginning to give confirmation.

Line of Light

Spiritual training at the outset can look unrealistic. It says: 'Do this!' or 'Don't do that!', but a bare command can defeat its own purpose. It is like the King in *Alice in Wonderland*, who angrily tells the trembling witness: 'Give your evidence. And don't be nervous. I'll have you executed if you're nervous!' There are some things that cannot just be commanded.

We feel that an order not to be nervous is like an order not to feel cold, or an order to like eating something unpleasant. The question is whether feelings can be controlled by a simple order, even when backed up with a threat of beheading.

In yoga the words used are more gentle; perhaps something on these lines:

> A student of yoga should do his actions without personal hopes or fears about the result.

But the point remains: how is this to be done in real life? To do it, one would have to be already free from hope and fear. Surely he would be a master, not a student.

Now, there is a central teaching in yoga:

> *A fundamental change in behaviour can normally be brought about only by changing the very roots of the mind, and not by changing just the surface ideas.*

To change the roots of the mind, namely the latent dynamic samskāra-impressions, needs sustained effort. It is true that there are some yogic short-term helps in an emergency, but the effect is temporary. The real change is like bringing someone who has neglected his health into a state of vigour and physical ease. It takes some six weeks to get any noticeable improvement, and six months for a big change. It will require a good three years of intensive training to convert a feeble body into a physical instrument equipped with energy, endurance and precision.

Inner training is similar. Serious yoga practice gives some result in six weeks – a brief unexpected feeling of independence and inner control; after six months there will be a significant change. If the practices are kept up with continued enthusiasm (not as drudgery, or dogged fulfilment of a pledge to oneself), in three years there will be a radical change at the roots of the mind. This does not mean an end to difficulties inner and outer, but they are now met with creative zest.

So when we are faced with a 'Don't be nervous!' situation, it is a bit late to hope that some yoga technique, recalled from a book or lecture and only now adopted, will give instant calm. It will not. A non-swimmer who falls overboard cannot expect to duplicate the movements of swimmers seen on television. He ought to have learnt to swim long ago.

Still, yoga does teach certain things which if practised even a little can help in crises. They are life-belts, and no substitute for learning to swim. There is not always a life-belt available. Even the best yogic practices are uncertain in their effect until they have been done steadily for a good time. How long it takes depends also on what sort of life the practiser has been leading.

The mathematician Dodgson (who wrote *Alice in Wonderland* under the pen-name Lewis Carroll) was a good observer of human behaviour. The description of the Hatter's nervous panic in front of the King shows him fidgeting with his hands and feet. Then he bites his teacup instead of the bread-and-butter.

In yogic terms, the prāṇa-s or life-currents of an agitated person go in a stream to the extremities: hands, feet and face. This dispersal can be corrected by bringing the attention to the central line of the body.

The Opening Practice

1. Sit in a meditation posture (as described on pages 77-79). Sit in relaxation. This does not mean complete relaxation: the body would collapse. It means to have no more tension than what is required to hold the posture. In time, the body maintains itself without conscious control. Good posture helps to open up to the vital cosmic force which runs through everything.
2. Bunch the fingers and press them for a few seconds on the abdomen just below the navel. Take them away, and then use the after-sensation to focus the mind there.
3. Now breathe in deeply, without strain. Feel that the breath is coming in at the navel, and rising in a column

of light up the centre line of the body; it reaches the spot between the eyebrows at the end of the breath. Of course the physical breath does not in fact come in at the navel. But an easy way to become aware of the central vital current is to associate it with the movement of breath. The action is something like drawing up milk through a straw; here it is drawing up light.

On the out-breath, visualization is dropped. Mind rests. Then with the next in-breath, make the visualization again.

4. Do this twenty-one times. Count on the fingers, or finger joints, or make twenty-one knots in a piece of string and use like a rosary. The breath should be deep and slow, but not strained. With facility, it lengthens naturally; the exercise can last six or seven minutes. But a record-breaking spirit is pointless.

The practice tranquilizes the body and mind, and opens them to divine cosmic currents. To know too much about the theory, however, is a disadvantage at the beginning. It generally disturbs practice.

The Line of Light

One of the main traditions, which Dr Shastri followed, recommends focussing attention on the central line of the body, from the navel circle to the forehead. It is a development of the previous exercise. In this more general practice, there is no movement of the attention, nor focussing on the breath.

Press a fingertip on the top of the forehead, and slide the fingertip down the front of the body. Pass it with light pressure between the brows, over the nose, chin, throat, breast, and end up at the navel. Use the after-sensation to bring the mind to the central line. Feel it as a line of calm light. Sit for ten minutes, looking at it, and feeling it. This is called the Line of Light practice, or in some traditions, the inner Middle Way.

Some experts add that in life situations when the impulse to move the body becomes very strong, the abdominal muscles (felt as being just below and round the navel) may be lightly tensed and then relaxed. Suppose you have to wait for a time before doing something active and important or even dangerous. Quite often the aimless tensing of muscles of hands and feet during the waiting period leads to loss of tone, so that when finally there is the relief of going into action, the movements come out jerky and poorly co-ordinated. Bringing the attention again and again to the central line, along with occasional tensing and relaxing the muscles felt to be round the navel, can prevent the loss of coordination. By this practice symptoms of nervousness are reduced. But unless it has been done in favourable circumstances for a good time, it will not show its true effect in unfavourable ones.

> A ten-yard plank, a foot wide, is laid on the floor. Anyone could walk along it without stepping off. Many could do it with their eyes shut. But if it is the foot-wide top of a high wall, few would like to try it. The task is the same, but the knowledge that one absolutely must not step off, makes the difference.

If a strong rail is provided on which the hand can rest, the walk is again manageable. Once a rail is there, it is not found necessary to clutch at it. Because it is there, it is not needed.

The application to life is, that the Line of Light becomes the strong rail.

It is practised first in a meditation situation. When some facility is attained, it can be done when waiting, walking, or at other times when the senses do not have to be continuously alert to the environment. Finally it will begin to rise, and support itself, without conscious effort of attention. When something upsetting happens, the Line of Light manifests itself as a protective and calming influence, and the inner balance is recovered. It is as natural a process as recovering physical balance in a sudden gust of wind. In these ways, a practiser becomes more and more independent of the opposites.

Some people complain of the difficulty of fixing the attention continuously. They have no difficulty in doing so when they watch a favourite TV serial, or try to pick up scandal from a conversation at the next table. For serious training, the attention is to be treated like a puppy. A long cord is attached to his collar; when he dashes off, his name is called and he is gently hauled in. He is made to sit by pushing his haunches down. Then the pressure is released, the command given, 'Away!' and he dashes off. Soon his name is called again, and he is gently but firmly dragged in and made to sit. It is important not to get angry and so frighten him. But he must be pulled in, or the point of the training is lost. After daily sessions for a week or so, he will begin to come in with joy when his name is called, and voluntarily stay till released. He accepts it as part of the pattern of life.

In something of the same way, the attention can be brought back to the Line, and after some practice, will stay there. The daily practice is, in one tradition, eight minutes.

For a long time, meditation, like all other forms of training, will have good days and bad days: sometimes it will be only 20 per cent successful, but sometimes 80 per cent. A lot depends on how the daily life is lived. If selfishness is reduced to some extent externally, it will not return to disturb the meditation. Then on certain days the meditator will become aware, not of a more-or-less selfish individual looking at light, but of being light, and catch a wondering glimpse of what he really is, beyond the mind-cage.

Karma-Yoga Action

In karma-yoga defined by Śaṅkara in II.39 commentary, there are three elements: (1) calm endurance of opposites, (2) yogic action, (3) samādhi practice. The first of these can be roughly summed up as Independence, and was looked at in a previous chapter. This chapter is concerned with the yogic action, from which karma-yoga takes its name.

Yogic action is presented, in the Gītā and in Śaṅkara, in slightly varying ways:

1. abandonment of, or evenness of mind towards, *results* good or bad;
2. dedicating, or consigning or depositing, *results* of actions, to God or Brahman;
3. dedicating, etc. the *actions* themselves to God or Brahman;
4. having no personal motive for actions;
5. giving up attachment to action as such;
6. giving up attachment to inaction.

It may be asked, why is inaction brought in? In the yogic analysis, even one sitting still, thinking 'Now let me be happily at ease', is still classed as acting. His choice is itself an action, and it soon changes. In a modem analogy, the safety catch has been put on, but the gun is still loaded and still in the hand. He is still a marksman.

The Gītā text mainly recommends actions based on traditional virtues such as those listed at the beginning of XVI: such actions are to be done without any personal motive of outer gain or recognition, or even inner self-satisfaction. Self-controlled action, uprightness, purity, and generosity are typical. It has been noticed how many of them consist in restraining one's own life, rather than direct interference with the lives of others. To set a good example of independence, and not injuring others, is most important in the Gītā ethics.

Apart from no greed for fruits, there is to be no attachment for action itself. Some people simply want to keep busy, without any personal interest in the particular results, though they often work hard. It is sometimes bossiness (as Dr Shastri remarked), but more often a way of asserting personal significance. It is not yogic action; it is motivated by a fear of becoming nothing.

> II.47 Your right must be to the action alone, never to its fruits;
> Let not the fruits of action be your motive, nor be attached to inaction.
>
> 48 Set in yoga perform your actions, casting off attachment; be the same in success or failure:
> This being-the-same is called Yoga.

If there is no motive of getting fruits, and one is not to lay any claim to the results of hard work, how will any action ever get started, let alone finished properly? Superficial reading of such texts can lead to superficial work. Some may feel that it means not to care whether one cleans the floor or not. Or if one does clean it, dirty patches can be left, because one is not supposed to be 'working for results'.

But this is not what the text says. It says: not to be attached to results, whether in anticipation as motive, or afterwards as some fruit; it does not say the work is not to be done. To leave dirty patches on the floor is not 'cleaning it without attachment to results': it is simply not cleaning the floor. A clean floor is not the 'fruit' of cleaning; it is the final stage of the operation itself. The fruit would be that others notice and appreciate it, or do not notice and immediately walk over it with muddy feet – a bad fruit. The yogin is to practise evenness of mind in both cases. In the second case, it is not a question of compressing the lips and saying nothing. Evenness of mind is an inner serenity that works hard but beyond that, does not care.

How can such things be achieved? It is a reasonable question. The answer is, that the skill has to be learnt by degrees, like any other skill. Yoga is skill in keeping the mind even. The yogic control of thought is first practised in everyday things: it is not a question of screwing oneself up to face grand successes or shattering disasters. At the beginning, the best practice occasions are simply physical jobs consisting of repetitive movements. What would normally be regarded as boring tasks, in fact. Cleaning or polishing largish surfaces, copy-typing, adding endless columns of figures, walking along a dimly-lit road on a dark night. These are favourable times for practising inner control.

Suppose there is a wide floor of stone squares to clean in about an hour. The cleaner makes a rough time-plan; then begins. When he is scrubbing one stone, a yogin does not think: 'This is the fifth one in the row; ten more to do here', and then 'nine more', 'eight more', up to 'Now the next row'. If some such thought comes up, he mentally throws it away. This is not too difficult to do, if he looks at the movement of the brush and begins to appreciate it. Similarly with irrelevancies like wondering what the others are doing, or wishing he were elsewhere, or memories, or anticipations. They drop away as he feels into the scrubbing movement.

One of the pleasures of the seaside is to watch the waves coming in, over or around a little rock or post. A small patch of foam is created, each time similar but with a slight difference. People can sit for a good time, enjoying the beauty and variety of the patterns. Now, the same thing is going on with the movements of the scrubbing brush, and as the scrubber enters into the movement, he begins to enjoy the beauty and variety of these patterns. The mind becomes serene, and the movements easier. As the natural texture of the stone shows itself, the worker can feel that something is being revealed in himself also. He moves on to the next stone, not with any feeling 'that's another one done', but as naturally as a new wave comes when the previous one has fulfilled itself.

If all goes well, he will one day feel that the brush is moving itself, so to say; it moves faster and more effectively. There is a unity of scrubber, scrubbing brush, soap-and-water, and stone. The senses become sharper: things are brighter, and there is a brightness within. When this happens, the state of samādhi is coming near.

> XIV.11 When all the gates of the senses radiate the light of knowledge,
> Then Sattva should be known to be asserting itself.

The above verse is a riddle to those who do not practise. The senses are both those of perception and those of action. When they begin to become radiant, things are seen as they are, not merely as means or obstacles to something else. Movements become lively but also precise and gentle. The effect is noticeable even in an aged or crippled body; just to see such a one working, gives inner peace.

Sometimes, however, a first experience creates excitement; mind is disturbed, personal egoism revives, and with it the feeling: 'This is mine, and I can do it again.' It may take months before the necessary freedom from attachment returns. But even one experience gives an insight into a secret of yogic action.

It is referred to in one of the short cryptic Gītā phrases:

> II.50 He whose mind is thus held in yoga of evenness, casts off here the vice or virtue of actions;
> Therefore devote yourself to yoga: *yoga is the art of skilful action.*

The last line is literally: 'in actions, yoga is skill (kauśalam).' The word kauśala means not only dexterity, capacity, and adroitness; it has also a sense of auspiciousness, benefit, things going well, and so on. It can mean something like a secret, as when it is said: 'the secret of politics is: good timing.' The translation as 'art' gives a hint at both senses. But here it refers to experiences in karma-yogic action; it is not a question of words.

As in the case of the opposites, the Gītā basically sets the aspiring yogin to find within himself the power to make efforts. 'Arise, and engage yourself in yoga' (IV.42). It is only later that the Gītā gives the methods of devotion to an external Lord for those who cannot yet find power within themselves. And as before, Śaṅkara softens the austerity of the instructions by recommending the karma-yogin to practise also devotion to the Lord. In the case of actions, it is to dedicate the actions, or the fruit of actions, to the Lord. True, the Gītā itself in III.30 has directed the karma-yogin to 'cast all actions on Me', but the 'Me' there refers to the supreme Self of the yogin. It is not till V.10 that the Gītā says 'setting all your actions in Brahman', which is repeated in XII.6 and XVIII.57, with the word 'casting' (saṃnyasya), namely renouncing. By Chapter XII, the devotional practice of the Gītā is in full flood, and Śaṅkara refers it back to karma-yoga from the beginning.

Dedication to the Lord makes it easier to become free from anticipations or fears connected with results. In a crisis, a subordinate faithfully carrying out the instructions of a respected superior feels inner relief; he has cast the responsibility for ultimate results on to the superior. Free from meaningless worry, his work becomes efficient.

In the field of yoga, depositing the actions or their fruits in devotion to the Lord makes the mind calm, and opens the possibility of seeing the Lord in the action itself.

Chapter XII.10 and 11 make a distinction between consigning actions to the Lord, and consigning their fruits. The first is to devote the whole life to a divine purpose: to move, eat and sleep for that alone. The second is to have worldly concerns for oneself and family and work for them also, but to be prepared to accept the results of those efforts as from the Lord. This too cannot be done except by practising yoga to some degree, as the text itself says.

The actions of the karma-yogin are aimed at thinning the veil hiding the divine. When action becomes purified of associations, there will be tiny glimpses of light in everyday routines.

Samādhi

The samādhi of karma-yoga is a method of tranquillizing the whole mental process, purifying the deep layers of the mind where the latent dynamic impressions lie, and focussing the stilled and purified mental energy on divine manifestations. Finally the higher mind is able to focus on the cosmic intelligence, the source of all manifestations. When such a mind comes to rest, time and space and body-consciousness forgotten, without even the thought 'I am meditating', the subject of meditation blazes forth in its own true nature: that is called samādhi.

The samādhi of the Gītā is not imagining as existent what does not exist. In the world, meditations can be used as auto-suggestions which can be helpful though not literally true. For instance, Japanese wrestlers, whose art consists mainly in pushing the opponent out of the ring, meditate: 'I am a great wave.' A champion attributed his success to practising this meditation, sometimes all night. He said that, in contest, he used to feel a mighty wave surging through him. In fact, the successful pushing action in these contests is a sort of wave movement.

On the other hand, Śaṅkara points out how, in ancient India, the central post in a ritual ceremony was meditated on as the sun. The splendour of the sun was felt to be in the post, and the ritualist was exalted. Still, he remained aware that the post is not actually the sun. Śaṅkara explains that in such cases the things continue to be known in the same way, and it is not supposed that there is a change of the substance. But he says repeatedly that the rituals do bring worldly success to those who perform them with full conviction.

In yoga, samādhi meditation is not directed at success in this or another world; such successes are illusory and create bonds. Nor is it any kind of exalting poetic simile. It can be compared to using a telescope to focus on something in a distant scene, not visible to the naked eye. The instrument is directed roughly in the right direction, and now the anticipated appearance of the sought object is vividly imagined. This is, it is true, an imaginary picture, but it is not wholly imaginary When something like it is dimly glimpsed, the telescope is held quite still, and focussed on it. Gradually the outline becomes clearer, and then the detail. It is not quite like what was imagined; but it is close enough to be recognized. Now it has become direct perception, not imagination. Similarly the mind has to be held steady in meditation, and then focussed on some aspect of the Lord. That aspect is first imagined from the classical descriptions given by those who have recorded their own experiments, but later directly perceived.

The first step, then, is tranquillization. It is first practised in a quiet place. Later, it has to be practised not only in retirement but in action, and when meeting the impact of the opposites. No one could call himself a swimmer who could swim only in perfectly still water, though certainly to break a world record, the water does have to be calm.

Some theory is necessary, but the main thing is practice. Without that, theories are sterile and disappointing.

> II.52 When your mind crosses the tangle of delusion
> You will get sick of all you have heard and all that they still want to tell you.

> 53 When your mind, turning from words, stands motionless, immovable in samādhi concentration,
> Then you will have attained yoga.

Samādhi practice, namely meditation in a secluded place, is the third element of karma-yoga. Later it will be compared to a candle burning steadily in a windless enclosure, and (by Śaṅkara) to a stream of oil smoothly pouring from a jar. In both the cases there is in fact movement: the flame is consuming the wax, the oil is passing down. But the successive states are so similar that it makes sense to say for instance that the flame does not move. Meditation aims first to make the successive states of the mind so similar that it does not appear to move.

The efforts in meditation towards samādhi can be explained in terms of waves, though as always the analogy must not be pressed too far. The first diagram represents a mixture of light waves of various wavelengths. Ordinary daylight is such a mixture.

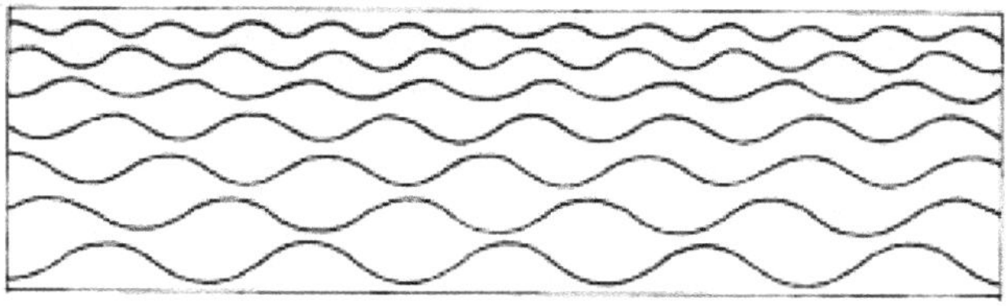

The next diagram shows waves all of the same wavelength. They would be seen as a pure colour, such as red.

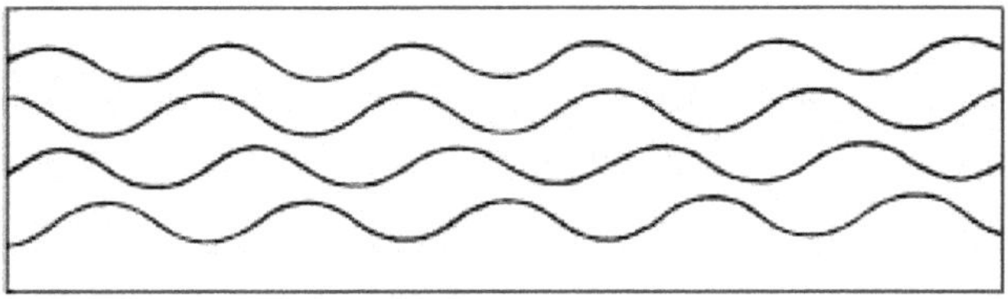

In the last diagram, the waves are not only all of exactly the same wavelength: they are 'coherent'. This is laser light, which can burn a hole in a steel plate in a few minutes.

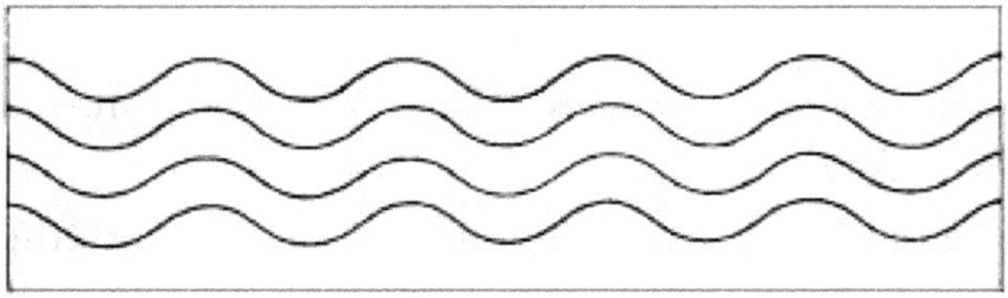

For some time, the mind in meditation is a mixture of thoughts; it is, so to say, mostly ordinary daylight. But by practice, a certain stream of thought is encouraged and finally becomes dominant. This can be done only by persisting with the same meditation, with interest and expectancy (not anxiety), for at least six weeks. When the thoughts are all on the same line, it is meditation. The successive thoughts are now similar. If this is continued, on the same object, thoughts become not merely similar but the same. They come to one point, and the mind is felt to stop on that point. This is samādhi. The awareness 'I am meditating on this' is thinned away, and the object alone remains, in a radiance. Up to this point, the meditation has had to be constantly supported; it was an idea in the mind. Now the object stands in its own strength; it is an experience of direct perception.

Such an experience, however, is not necessarily a clear revelation of truth; it is usually mixed up with latent impressions of words and ideas from the depths of the mind. These distort it. But if the process is repeated daily, they begin to drop away, and the divine energy and light are realized as pouring through, and upholding, what has been meditated on.

As meditation progresses, there is an increasing awareness of space: it is called, in the ancient Upaniṣad-s, 'the space within the heart'. The object may be seen shining in a vast space. It does not do to give many descriptions. The mind may build them into some detailed expectation, and then use that individual mental construct as a touchstone. The genuine experience, on the other hand, when it comes, is always a surprise: the meditator for the first time really understands what the ancient texts refer to. They appear in a new light, and confirm what has happened.

There are later confirmations of knowledge and power, in what is loosely called inspiration. In the scientific field we can look at Becquerel's discovery of radioactivity (in darkness, when he was looking for X-rays produced by fluorescent light), or Rutherford's crucial experiment in 1911 which gave the clue to atomic structure. We find that the decisive action was taken contrary to the whole logic of the situation. It was not chance: the discoveries resulted from their own illogical actions. They were impelled, almost like marionettes, to seemingly quite irrational behaviour. The result in each case was amazing. Rutherford emphasizes this in his account. He led a dedicated life, exceptionally free from worldly considerations, he despised money. His genius inspired two generations of physicists. He was a yogin of science, and used to say that he felt a unity with the newly discovered alpha-particles: 'I feel I know what they are going to do.'

Inspiration comes as a result of prolonged concentration; the divine breath is attracted, and then struggles to express itself through the limited channel of the individual mind. It thus varies in quality of expression, depending on the clarity and purity of the receiving channel. Children may hear a lecture on cosmology, or hear a Beethoven sonata: how much they get from it depends on how far their minds have developed in the fields of physics or music.

Relations revealed by physics are only a tiny part of the divine manifestation. In the ultimate analysis, they are illusory. Scientists are no more fulfilled than others: artists may be better off, since their earlier work is not necessarily replaced by later. Shakespeare is still read by millions, but not Newton. The yogin has to penetrate much deeper than a scientist or an artist.

Chapters VII–X of the Gītā give subjects for meditation by karma-yogins. Śaṅkara stresses at the beginning of VII that it is not a question of building emotional faith and stopping there. It must lead to direct vision in samādhi, vision which pierces the veils of differences. It is true that if anything at all is meditated on steadily for a long time, the divine will shine from it. But the seen world is like a great desert, under which there is known to be water; some places are easier to dig, and some are rocky and refractory. So the Gītā recommends certain classes of things as most suitable for practice.

One is the essential characteristics of a thing, for instance, the heat and brilliance of fire. In the human sphere, the Lord is austerity in the ascetics, intelligence in the intelligent, heroism of the heroes. When a man sees such things in others, or finds a trace of them in himself, he meditates: 'This is not an individual possession: it is from the Lord.' After some time, the roots of the mind begin to change. He becomes free from jealousy at seeing these things in others, and free from arrogance when they manifest in himself. And that is a great relief: some have said it is like getting out of a room in which there is a snake concealed somewhere.

Another type of meditation is on the Lord as the highest manifestation in some class. 'Of mountains, I am Himālaya ... of animals the lion ... of words, 'I am the sacred syllable OM.' There are many examples frxom Indian traditional history: 'I am Rāma of warriors, ... of rivers, the Ganges', and other such which mean little to the West. The scope becomes wider: 'I am the origin of all beings ... Of the feminine I am Fame, Fortune, Speech, Memory, Understanding, Constancy, Patience.' All these words are feminine in Sanskrit grammar, but Śaṅkara points out that prosperity has always been symbolized as a goddess, and that the virtues given are characteristic of women at their best.

The list has been mainly of what is regarded by human beings as favourable, but it begins to include what they feel as darker: 'Of the trickster, I am the dice', loaded, we may assume. 'I am all-seizing death.' Then again, previously it had been said: 'I am the desire that is not opposed to righteousness', but now comes also, 'I am desire.' This meditation does not mean that wrong desires should be yielded to; they are to be opposed by the yogin. As he stands, they are his enemies, and so the Gītā has termed them in III.37–43. But through this meditation, he takes one more step, and sees them not as enemies but as opponents. They are like fellow wrestlers in the training hall, against whom he struggles with all his skill and endurance, but without hating or fearing them. They have been selected and pitted against him by the Trainer. In combat with them, he builds up good physique, balance and speed, strength of will and general health. This example was sometimes given by Dr Shastri; wrestling is a national sport in India, and one of his fellow disciples was a champion amateur wrestler.

The final meditation of the karma-yogin is the universal form of the Lord partially described in Chapter XI.

Here is a short account of samādhi experience by Dr Shastri's own teacher, in his book *The Heart of the Eastern Mystical Teaching*. It is given in a context of yoga practice of self-control and devotion to the Lord:

> If you meditate daily in this way for eighteen months and every now and then devote a week or two entirely to it, you will, in your meditation, lose consciousness of both the world and yourself and experience only the object of meditation. You will see an extraordinary light resembling the colour of a lotus, in its intensified form, in your heart and all mental limitations will disappear. This state is called samādhi.

Again, he says of meditation:

> The feeling that I am not the body is the primary condition of the Yoga, and the complete relinquishment of body-consciousness marks the attainment of samādhi.
>
> While you have consciousness of time and space you will not see Ātman.

The state passes. But by repeating it, the dynamic seed-impressions forming the basis of the mind are purified, and become partially transparent. Then the vision of the Lord is still seen, as if through a thin veil, during ordinary active life. The Gītā calls this state also, by extension, samādhi. But it generally uses the word as defined in the passage above. In the pure samādhi, the veil of body-consciousness is not merely thinned, but completely withdrawn. Dr Shastri quoted St Paul of 2 Corinthians 3:18: 'But we with face unveiled behold as in a mirror the Lord, and are changed into the same image, from glory to glory reflecting.'

Purity of Being (Sattva-śuddhi)

When the three elements of karma-yoga have been practised for a long time, or a shorter time with more intensity, things become simpler. Independence of the opposites, acting in evenness of mind, and samādhi-meditations on aspects of the Lord, produce an inner peace and energy. Life becomes like walking over open countryside towards a clear objective, instead of being lost in crowded streets, assailed by tricksters, beggars, tempters, shouters, and radios at full blast.

In this connection, Dr Shastri sometimes used the simile of electricity to give students an idea of the practice:

> Don't act so much that your soul will be tired, and don't be so fond of solitude that you do not fulfil the reasonable expectations of the world. Man charges his being with spiritual electricity, and discharges that electricity by means of his thoughts and by means of his actions. The soul has to be charged every day with divine spiritual electricity, otherwise it will all be spent. And when it is about to be spent entirely, you feel worried, melancholic, with inclinations to

> suicide, and so on. These are the symptoms that it is nearing exhaustion. ... You have to charge your battery every day. How? In silence, meditation, holy study ... for at least two hours a day. If you properly meditate, not as a burden, not as a pledge fulfilled, your soul will be healthy and you will not be a victim to boredom, melancholy, over-sensitiveness and the like. The electricity is generated in the alchemy of your soul: bring your mind nearer and nearer to the great Self. Withdraw your mind from the objects of the senses, from the world, from love and hate: bring it nearer to OM, and rest there, and it will be charged. Then when you act, you act as a karma-yogin, and your actions will be perfect.

When the interior clamour has died down to a considerable extent, the state is called Purity of Being. The karma-yogin begins to be attracted to the Knowledge texts. Though Arjuna could not yet undertake the Knowledge-yoga, which requires an experience of the Self to enter it, still texts on the Self were given to him from the very beginning: 'Eternal, present everywhere, fixed, immovable is He, the Self' (II.24).

While the mind is completely enmeshed in individual considerations, this is nonsense. How can my self – even with a capital letter, Self – be present everywhere? It is clearly confined in the body. At most, these phrases could be somehow poetical, perhaps symbolic of man's infinite aspiration – so says the mind entangled in limitations.

With karma-yoga practice, mind finds itself less cluttered. Thinking and feeling become spaced out, and through the gaps there are glimpses of a light which is not the light of perception or conception. The Knowledge texts begin to pull.

Even so, it seems incredible. 'I am that all-pervading divine Self': the mind draws back before such a text. Here teachers recommend meditation on bare 'I am'. Mind tries to complete this with 'I am British', 'I am Chinese', 'I am man', 'I am woman', 'I am young', 'I am old'. All these are to be rejected. 'No, no. I am, I am, I am.' We think we know 'I am', but we know it only as 'I am here, I am not there, I am thinking, I am remembering', and so on. It is possible to dismiss these adjuncts, as Śaṅkara calls them; they are no more the Self than clothes are their wearer.

When 'I am' meditation comes to maturity, that is to say has laid down saṃskāra-impressions of truth in the depths of the being, 'I am' will be completed in a living awareness of the true I. This is called Knowledge; the yogin who has purified his being by karma and samādhi, in time finds it in himself by himself (IV.38). The Lord within stirs and shows himself. When this happens, the path of Knowledge begins.

'I am' is an actor throwing off the props which identify his role. The play King takes off his heavy crown. Long John Silver lays down his crutch; in the play, he cannot walk without it, but now he moves around to stretch his legs. He takes it up again when he is to go back to his role, but for the moment, he wants to be free of it. Similarly, during the meditation period, the karma-yogin is, so to speak, stretching himself and then sitting in the wings.

On a special occasion for a special divine purpose, he might throw off the restrictions of the role even during the performance of the play. When Jesus is arrested, the Fourth Gospel describes him as asking: 'Who is it you want?' to which the police reply: 'Jesus of Nazareth.' Then he says: 'I am.' At his 'I am', they recoil and fall to the ground. Translators, Western and Eastern, amend it to 'I am he', because 'I am' would not fit in with the scene. It has to be 'I am someone or something', otherwise it does not make sense to the world. But perhaps at that moment the star of the play threw off momentarily his role of defenceless ascetic, and exposed the other actors, powerful in the play, as very little in reality. Then as though recollecting himself, and setting up the play again, he repeats his first question: 'Who is it you want?' They make the same reply: 'Jesus of Nazareth', and now he picks up the script, as it were: 'I have told you that I am – if I am the man you want, let these others go free.'

The main function of the I Am meditation is to discard the make-up and conviction of the reality of the role. The true status is then apparent without striving: in the realization of Brahman there is no effort, says Śaṅkara.

'Well, even so [the mind raises its endless objections], how could that true status be the one all-pervading Lord? The analogy does not hold: the actors are still separate. We may have unsuspected depths, but we are still different selves. It is obviously so. All the spiritual sales talk cannot alter that. One individual is very limited physically and mentally: there is not very much to him or her. Whereas another is gifted and energetic and ambitious, and thus very effective in the world. How can they be called the same?' So objects the mind.

The tradition answers: 'The analogy was a sign-post. It must not be taken beyond the point it is meant to illustrate. What you call sales talk is to help a wavering mind to keep to the practice; one that can really take decisions would not need it. I give you another, for your new question. But the question can be finally settled only by experience, not by analogies or inferences or guesses.

Under great deserts like Sahara or Thar, there are equally great sheets of water. Sometimes there are underground streams. This was known in very early times. The communities set about digging wells, some large and some small. The ancients dug wells over 1,000 feet deep. As a well got deeper, groundwater would appear in it. This might vary very much. A well could have a limited capacity; in some seasons it might dry up. These wells were indeed separate from each other, with different capacities.

But if it went deep enough to reach an underground river, the well could never be exhausted. Whether its diameter was great or small, the water supply was unlimited. So though such wells had different locations, they were now all one – the underground stream. A tiny well might have room for only one bucket. But when that bucketful had been taken, the well would still be full.

The stream of divine inspiration can come through the channel of a brilliant intellect, strong will, and widely recognized charity: but it also comes through an illiterate, slow-thinking and obscure channel. The teacher of St Anselm was Lanfranc, also one of the great minds of the Middle Ages, and also Archbishop of Canterbury to the early Norman dynasty in England. His own teacher, who inspired this subtle Italian ex-lawyer with vision and purity of purpose, had been Herlwin, an almost illiterate hermit monk.

Śāriputra was one of the Buddha's chief disciples; he became so famous that some early texts of other schools speak of him as the Buddha himself: Śāriputra the Buddha. He had previously been head of another sect, but was converted to Buddhism, without any words being spoken. He saw Ajita, one of the first followers of the Buddha, walking in the street on a begging round. He went up to him and said: "From the way you walk, I am somehow sure that you have solved the riddle of existence. Teach me." Ajita replied: "My teacher is now staying on the hill called Vulture Peak: you will recognize it from the black and white rocks, like a vulture's feathers. Ask him." This incident is all that is recorded of Ajita. But it changed the spiritual history of India and of much of the rest of Asia.

While the well is self-sufficient, it has identity. "I am large", "I am small", "My water is sweet", "My water alas is briny". But when the digging has gone down to the deep river, there is no more separate identity, only the rush of the river: "I am, I am, I am."'

Knowledge

When karma-yoga practice – endurance of the opposites, samādhi practice, and performance of actions in evenness of mind – has purified the basis of the yogin's being, Knowledge arises. Sometimes it is said that the Lord gives the Knowledge; sometimes that the Lord in the heart lights the flame of Knowledge, sometimes that Knowledge comes naturally. The difference in expression depends on how far the Lord is still regarded as external and apart.

Although the word knowledge has to be used for the Sanskrit word jñāna, it is not an exact equivalent. Knowledge in English means knowledge-of-something. In the phrase Knowledge Is Power, the first word means having objective information, for instance, a secret. But jñāna can also mean what we could only call pure Awareness, irrespective of any object. When it is occasionally said that Brahman is Knowledge Absolute, it points to awareness beyond the dualities of mind processes.

The form of the Knowledge is first a Self-realization, the thought: 'Here I am, free, without agency or actions or results; there is none other than 1.' This removes the restricted and illusory worldly idea: 'There are many things, and among them I move and I act aiming at this or that result.' This last has been an absolute conviction, and to remove it there has to be the absolute conviction of the thought of the true universal Self. The Self-realization must be as complete and immediately experienced as the previous immediately experienced bondage. It cannot come about unless the present unconscious convictions of the reality of the world are dissolved.

Then the conviction is: 'I am Brahman.' This is, however, still a thought. Even highest Knowledge is still a thought like other thoughts; it is an illusion supported on pure consciousness. The Truth-thought destroys other illusions, and then itself also, leaving pure consciousness, called supreme Self. Self-realization is sometimes loosely referred to as Freedom; but Freedom is not a process at all. Supreme Self is ever free, and has nothing to do with ideas of binding or freeing. The point comes up again and again. The path continues till thought is transcended. Brahman has no need to think. In reality, there is no second thing for it to think. Dr Shastri wrote: 'In the Vedānta of holy Śaṅkara, the disciplined and tranquillized mind can reflect glimpses of the Self Absolute, but the mind can under no condition whatsoever reveal the nature of the Self as truth-consciousness-bliss.'

Knowledge arises when the unconscious reservations about the truth begin to dissolve. What are these reservations? The holy texts declare that the Lord is everywhere, and this is confirmed by samādhi on divine manifestations. But there is an unconscious reservation: 'Yes, everywhere. But not *here*.' The texts say that the Lord is the life in all beings. This too is accepted and partially confirmed, but again with a reservation: 'But not in *me*.'

When the reservations go, Knowledge arises as the conviction: 'I am Brahman.' Though still a thought, this thought undermines the first part of itself. The 'I', a limited, individual, ever personally motivated and acting, apparent self, loses these local characteristics which seem to rule it off within Brahman. It disappears as such: Brahman remains in infinite majesty and glory, as it always was.

How is it possible? In his commentary to Chapter XIII Śaṅkara meets the numerous objections of the philosophers of the time. A commentator had to do this in order to be accepted; it was part of the intellectual tradition so strong in Indian culture. Many of his detailed refutations are no longer relevant today. But he gives also more direct and simple arguments. One is, the case of one who wrongly supposes he has eaten poison. The mere idea can actually kill him, as Śaṅkara says.

In some Japanese research on such cases, X-ray photographs showed intestinal spasms, accompanied by pain. If the doctor succeeds in convincing the patient, however, the latter can realize: 'I the sick patient, was never in fact sick. 'I have always been well.'

This realization, like the realization, 'I thought I was in Ignorance, but I have always been Brahman', undermines its first part. 'I the sick patient' is destroyed, not only in the present but in the past also. 'I am not sick, and have never been sick.' There remains only: 'I have always been well.'

For a short time, the sight of the hospital bed and nurse and doctor may vividly recall the imagined illness. Again, if the child of a neighbour brings some flowers for the sufferer, it would be tactless to say: 'Oh, I have never been sick, I don't need those.' The patient would continue to play the part, and thank her gratefully.

While still passionately involved in events great or small, it is very difficult to imagine the state of Knowledge. Small children boast of what they will do when grown-up. They dream of having size and strength, property and money. But these things are then used for childish purposes. Children cannot take it in when told: 'You won't want to buy lots of toys when you're grown-up.' They cannot imagine themselves sitting, as their parents do now, just talking endlessly with friends.

In the same way, when an attempt is made to conceive the rise of Knowledge in some saint, qualities like universality are readily accepted. But immediately afterwards, the God-realized one is spoken of as 'he' or 'she'. Properly speaking, after I am Brahman there is no he or she; there remains only an illusory body-mind complex which is, as it were, a finger of Brahman. It is not a personal individual existence, revolving round itself. But the habit of personification is so ingrained in an unillumined mind, that however much it may be denied, personification at once returns. The universal Self is stuffed back into a human body, in the imagination of the unillumined people. The holy texts recognize this, and do provisionally allow name and personality to the illumined. Otherwise an aspirant would hardly be able to think at all about Brahman-realization. But the Gītā takes care to show that it is the Lord who manifests in what seems to be a sage: 'Of priests I am Bṛhaspati ... of great sages I am Bhṛgu ... of divine sages I am Nārada ... of Vṛṣṇi clansmen I am Vāsudeva (Kṛṣṇa) ... of ascetics I am Vyāsa, of the wise, I am wise Uśanas.'

The same point comes repeatedly. The Gītā declares:

> XV.19 He who undeluded thus knows Me, the supreme Spirit, (as I am He,)

He knows all, and his whole thought is on Me.

It is said that he knows the supreme Spirit as 'I am He' (this is Śaṅkara's expansion of the original word 'thus'). Then, He knows all, he is omniscient. This is sometimes taken to mean that he ought to know what is happening on the other side of the world, in detail.

Sometimes a teacher will ridicule the supposition. It rests on the idea that after realizing 'I am the supreme Spirit', somehow a 'he' has been crammed back into the surviving body-mind complex. Then (it is concluded) that body-mind ought to be omniscient, because the text says so. Such a 'man' ought never to need a railway time-table; he should know already the times of all trains. That is the illogical supposition.

Śaṅkara anticipates this misconception, which must have been equally common in his day. It is not the body-mind that knows all about things at a distance, but the universal Self which knows everything because it *is* everything, being the Self of all. As having entered its own illusory projections, Brahman is everything: including trains, time-tables, and body-minds of limited worldly knowledge.

The texts sometimes say that we all have true Knowledge all the time, but awareness of it is masked by our obsession with objects, whether external or internal. Internal objects include mind and ego and dynamic latent tendencies: they are not Self. A clue is given in the Kena Upaniṣad: 'What the mind cannot think, but by whose power the mind thinks, know that to be Brahman, and not what the people worship as apart.'

As an example from life: a short-sighted man cannot find his glasses. A humorous friend comes in as he is searching a cluttered table, and says: 'Why, you're looking at them.' The searcher redoubles his efforts, 'Not there.' He tries the floor. 'You're still looking at them,' repeats the friend. 'But I've searched everywhere now.' 'What are you searching with – a short-sighted man like you?' 'What do you mean?' 'Give up looking for them; shut your eyes and *feel.*' Now he feels the glasses on his nose. What his eyes could not see, yet by whose power the eyes were seeing, that was the glasses. Afterwards he was aware of them as enabling him to see: in a way he then sees them, though not seeing them.

There is some parallel with the case of Knowledge. Turning away from objects, closing the eyes and feeling, could be a hint for samādhi. Afterwards, there is awareness of a light behind the mind, whose awareness was masked by the obsession with objects. The light is the bliss of Brahman-knowledge:

> VI.28 The yogin who has held to yoga, freed from taint,
> Easily attains contact with Brahman, the endless bliss.
>
> 29 He sees himself as in all beings, and all beings in himself...
>
> 30 He sees Me, the Lord, in all, and all in Me.

Samnyāsa – Throwing Off Action

It was expected, as a natural result of the Knowledge 'I am Brahman', that the surviving body-mind complex would continue to move for a time under its own momentum. Śaṅkara gives the example of the arrow.

In medieval times, a battlefield message could be sent by binding it round an arrow, which was then shot to land in front of the intended recipient. If, after it was released, a sudden event made the message unnecessary, or even misleading, the arrow would still inevitably go on to complete its course. If however it had not yet been shot, though already on the string, it would be quietly replaced in the quiver. The illustration is given by Śaṅkara in his Gītā commentary. After God-realization, those actions which have already begun to produce their effects – already in the air, so to speak – will go on till their force is spent; but new actions will normally not be initiated.

It was called saṃnyāsa: throwing away, or discarding or renouncing or giving up, action. Translations like 'renouncing', 'giving up', 'abandoning' do not do full justice to the word. Renunciation and giving up often have a sense of reluctance;

people give up in despair, or renounce their rightful claims. But saṃnyāsa is a compound, from 'sam' complete, 'ni' down, 'as' to cast. It means a complete throwing down as a voluntary, natural and joyful act. Though itself an action, it ends action. Just so when a king signs the act of abdication, which ends his royal power, it is itself an exercise of that power, though for the last time. The formal act of saṃnyāsa, which involved leaving home and all connections, would correspond to an act of abdication. In classical times formal saṃnyāsa meant life as a mendicant, distinguished sometimes by a coarse orange robe, neither attached to bodily life nor seeking bodily death. To see such walking symbols of absolute freedom, dependent on nothing, often gives courage to people of the world in distress. The Gītā describes them as usually wandering, though monasteries were allowed; Śaṅkara himself founded some important ones which still flourish. Those who practise the life say it is a very healthy one, and some attain a vigorous old age. In his commentary to Gītā XVIII.3 Śaṅkara points out that those who have seen the Self, and are on the path of Knowledge (jñāna-niṣṭhā), do not find in the Self any pain at all arising from physical conditions; and there are no inner anxieties at all.

The previous life was karma-yoga in the world, energetically acting but free from selfish entanglements of attachment or fear. Without much inner friction, it will have been efficient and a success, spiritually and often socially as well. The gradual purification of the inner being takes a good time, and usually the karma-yogin will have fulfilled his social role by the time Knowledge rises in him. When, as a result of the inner clarity, he 'finds Knowledge in himself by himself' (IV.38), there is a natural impulse to hand over his social role to those now due to undertake it. Classically, before seeking liberation, the Three Debts must be repaid. One of them was the debt to the 'ancestors'; the term included the society which brought one up. Just so it would be only after a hardworking reign that the king could properly abdicate in favour of his heir.

As previously explained, a king is chosen as exemplar because he was the hardest-working and most responsible man in the kingdom: he had an eighteen-hour day, and no holidays. The principles apply to all who have responsibilities, in other words, to practically everyone.

Now suppose (as Śaṅkara suggests) that the king has personally initiated many important projects, which will still need him as a figurehead to get firmly established. Or suppose that neighbouring kings could seize the chance of a young inexperienced heir to make raids. In such cases, the ministers might ask the king to stay on for a time. They will run the country as he has trained them, but his mere presence will be a centre for the enthusiasm and loyalty of the whole people.

In yogic terms, Śaṅkara allows that in such cases the natural course for the surviving body-mind of the man of Knowledge would be to remain in the world. The Self does not act, but the ministers – body, senses, active mind – act as they have been trained by the karma-yoga discipline. The higher mind should remain in a current of: 'I do nothing at all.' So the throwing off of action is here internal.

> V.13 Mentally giving up all actions, he sits happily, presiding over the city of nine gates,
> Never at all acting, nor causing to act.

The ministers, namely body, senses and lower mind, continue acting out the programmes initiated before Knowledge; the thoughts and actions are almost entirely of sattva. They do not initiate new programmes; there is no individual will or purpose any more to do so. It is a running down of the sattvic impulses already in operation.

However the Gītā points out, and Śaṅkara confirms, that the Lord may himself move such a body-mind as part of his cosmic purpose: it becomes an instrument, a finger, moved by another. Then normal expectations and limitations are transcended in an uprush of divine knowledge and power, sometimes concealed and sometimes revealed. Dr Shastri once remarked that one of the pleasures of chess is when one side has sacrificed nearly everything, but manages to checkmate with a remaining pawn. He said that there are spiritual lessons to be learnt from chess. Both sides appreciate the seeming miracle of the lone pawn, and then the pieces are gathered up, bits of wood with all distinctions gone, and put away in the box. The two former opponents look at each other and smile.

Knowledge-Stance: Jñāna-Niṣṭhā

Following on Right Knowledge of the identity of the true Self and Brahman, Śaṅkara presents two more means to release, though they are really stages in clarity of Knowledge: (1) saṃnyāsa or casting away action, (2) what he calls jñāna-niṣṭhā, or Standing on Knowledge. Strictly speaking, they are both corollaries, natural results, of Right Knowledge; but he often treats them separately.

Saṃnyāsa has been discussed already; it is the inner living realization that the Self does not act. In the case of those who have already fulfilled their role, it is reflected outwardly in withdrawal from active life; for others, sattvic action of the body-mind complex (not the Self), continues as long as life lasts.

Now look at what Śaṅkara says about jñāna-niṣṭhā. Jñāna means knowledge: it comes from jñā, a remote relative of the English 'know'. Niṣṭhā comes from a verb sthā, to stand firmly. The sense is, that the Brahman-Knowledge has to be under the feet as well as in the head. As several Upaniṣad-s say, it must give strength. While it is in the head alone, it is still only an idea, one among many.

Sometimes jñāna-niṣṭhā is translated 'devotion to knowledge'. However, devotion is usually towards what one is not, or has not; devotion to the king is felt by subjects, not by the king himself. Śaṅkara's Gītā commentary does not use jñāna-niṣṭhā to mean a yearning for Knowledge. Rather it is total immersion in Knowledge already attained. Niṣṭhā usually means firm establishment: Brahma-niṣṭhā refers to a spiritual teacher established in Brahman; japa-niṣṭhā is one constantly engaged in japa or repetition of a mantra; tapo-niṣṭhā is one wholly taken up with tapas, austerity-meditation. It must be remembered that phrases like 'establishment of Knowledge' are tentative. It is not that the Knowledge itself becomes dim or wavers; but that it seems to be dimmed, as the sun seems to be dimmed by clouds, or seems to waver when reflected in a rippling stream, or seems to move along above a runner.

Jñāna-niṣṭhā is taking a firm stand on Knowledge. It is not a search for some new purely intellectual insight; it is not affirming an idea or theoretical notion. Sometimes Śaṅkara calls it samyag-darśana-niṣṭā, establishing right vision, or ātma-darśana-niṣṭhā, establishing vision of Self. These words are very strong in Śaṅkara's vocabulary: they mean direct awareness, as immediate as a sense experience. They never mean an idea unsupported by experience.

What would it be in practice, this Jñāna-niṣṭhā, standing on Knowledge or Knowledge-stance? An example has been given previously about air travel. There are intelligent and well informed people who will not travel by air. Friends show them the figures, which they agree are convincing: yet they continue to refuse. They have correct knowledge, but illusion persists, at least for a time. If they make the effort to think it through again and again, the illusion weakens and finally drops away. They can then stand on their knowledge, and go by air when they need to.

In the case of Brahman-Knowledge, Śaṅkara often lists stages. In his commentary to V.12 he gives them as (1) karma-yoga, (2) purification of the inner being, (3) attainment of Knowledge (jñāna-prāpti), (4) Casting Off Action (saṃnyāsa), (5) jñāna-niṣṭhā or Knowledge-stance, and finally (6) Freedom (mokṣa). Sometimes he abbreviates the list. Either Casting Off Action, or alternatively jñāna-niṣṭhā, can stand for both of them taken together. Sometimes he says simply: 'Knowledge is the means to Freedom.' This is not a contradiction of the full list: the rest is implied. In the same way, a potential refugee might be told: 'We'll be waiting at the frontier; all you have to do is get there.' It is not quite all; for instance, he must arrive secretly. But that is implied.

Again, when Śaṅkara says, as he so frequently does: 'Knowledge is the means to freedom', or 'Knowledge is the cause of Freedom', Knowledge here has its basic meaning: absolutely clear Knowledge free from memory-shadows of illusion. The words for 'means' (upāya) and 'cause' (kāraṇa) are the ordinary ones for something that brings about something else. Knowledge, in so far as it is still a mental conviction mixed up with memories of other things, is not itself Freedom. But when it has completely destroyed the world-illusions, it is the means to instant Freedom. Finally it will have destroyed itself too, as an idea.

The opponent repeatedly objects: 'If Knowledge is the means to Freedom, why the mention of stages like Casting Off Action, and Standing On Knowledge? Knowledge alone should produce the Freedom.'

His reply, given in a number of places, is, that these *are* Knowledge. They may be needed because it can happen that past involvements with the world, entered into before Knowledge arose, have left traces in the depths of the mind which can disturb the pure stream of Knowledge. Even after enlightenment by Knowledge, the mind of a sage may be affected by them. Jñāna-niṣṭhā, standing on Knowledge, is the effort to restore the natural clear stream of Self-Knowledge.

'Oh,' says the opponent triumphantly, 'then the man of Knowledge is subject to disturbances from the world just like an ordinary man. He is not free at all. So how could one have confidence in the process of Self-realization as a means to freedom? If he too has to make efforts at jñāna-niṣṭhā, he cannot have realized his true Self, which he is supposed to have done already. He must be still subject to illusions.'

The argument is strong, and Śaṅkara gives it in its full force in order to meet it convincingly. First of all, his answer may be summarized:

> Even after attainment of Knowledge, the mind may be disturbed by vivid memories of passionate worldly associations. But though they disturb, they are known to be unreal. The effort of jñāna-niṣṭhā is not to produce or reinforce Knowledge, but to dissipate memories of the unreal which in some cases may persist for a time.

There are three cases of inner disturbance to consider: the untrained man of the world, the karma-yogin who is training, and the Knower. Of these, the untrained man of the world, and the karma-yogin who is training, see the world as real. Both of them are upset by its changes. But the karma-yogin is making efforts to purify and still his inner being, and is beginning to have glimpses of the Lord behind the worldly appearances. He soon recovers his balance, whereas the man of the world merely tries to manipulate it to improve his personal situation.

Their minds throw up disturbances based on impressions of passionate entanglements of the past: 'If I had done that, I should have been rich now', 'that was delightful, and perhaps it could happen again', 'that was a terrible threat, and how can I avoid it?' 'Oh, this world ....'. The yogin tries to calm his mind, especially by devotion to God. He tries to see the divine hand in what happens; he goes into meditation to discover what his own role should be.

The man of Knowledge was just like the others before he attained it. He has come to know, now, that the threats and promises, hope and despair, were all based on unreal things, and were unreal themselves. They were stage props in the cosmic drama. Still, they recur, spontaneously remembered like scenes from a play seen formerly, known to be unreal, yet still with some power to move. The obstructions and disturbances are cleared away by effort: they are unreal, unreal, unreal. But there is no effort in the Knowledge itself. This is a key point to remember when looking at Śaṅkara's brief definitions of jñāna-niṣṭhā. For example, he says: 'jñāna-niṣṭhā is an intent effort to establish a continuous current of the idea of the transcendent Self'. It does not mean forcibly reviving and continuously reinforcing the Knowledge-current; it is a shorthand phrase for removing obstructions and distractions to that current which flows on naturally after Knowledge has been attained.

Again and again the point comes up: how can there be any real obstruction by what is known to be unreal? Again and again the Gītā itself says that there can:

> II.60 The impetuous senses rush off with the mind of an aspirant even though he knows them for what they are.
>
> III.39 By this, in the forms of desire, is obscured the Knowledge of even the one who knows;
> It is his constant enemy, and an insatiable fire.

While the body lasts, upheld by the impetus of past actions done before God-realization, there is a shadow-centre of personality remaining. As long as it still finds itself disturbed by past memories, it practises jñāna-niṣṭhā.

There are accounts of jñāna-niṣṭhā practice in a number of Gītā passages. Typical is XVIII.51–53:

> 51 With purified mind fixed in yoga, and firmly self-controlled,
> Throwing off sense-objects like sound, and putting away desire and aversion,
>
> 52 Living alone, eating little, restraining speech and body and mind,
> Ever engaged in one-pointed meditation on the Self, cultivating dispassion,
>
> 53 Without I-ness, straining, pride, desire, anger, possessiveness,
> – Free, unselfish, calm – he is ready to become Brahman.

Other passages are II.55–72, V.16–29. The central themes are: throwing away ties of the world, thus allowing the natural current of Self-realization to continue.

In some passages there are references to jñāna-niṣṭhā practised by those shadow-selves still seemingly strongly involved in the world by past unillumined actions and promises. V.8, 9 and 13 describe them as walking and talking, and in fact performing 'all actions'. But the seeming doer is to meditate in samādhi: 'I do nothing at all.' His samādhi, practised in the solitude of meditation, spreads out over the whole life.

jñāna-niṣṭhā is often called by Śaṅkara the supreme devotion to God: it is the devotion of the Knower. VII.16 speaks of four kinds of virtuous men who worship the Lord: one in danger, the seeker of worldly success, the seeker of Knowledge, and the Knower. Of them the Knower, practising yoga and devoted to the Lord alone, is highest:

> VII.18 All of them are noble, but the Knower I declare to be my very Self;
> Set in yoga, he turns to Me alone as the supreme goal.

Śaṅkara explains this as the supreme devotion (bhakti), as compared with the devotion of the other three, for whom the Lord is apart from themselves. He says that this Knower, set in yoga, is centred on the thought 'I myself am the Lord, I am none else'. In this way he strives to reach the Lord, concludes the great commentator.

One can feel it to be inconsistent, indeed absurd. How can one who already knows he is the Lord yet strive to reach the Lord? How can one have devotion to oneself? (This critical point is discussed at great length, in the Indian intellectual style, in Śaṅkara's commentary to XIII.2, but the intricacies there are not much help to a Western reader unfamiliar with the classical Indian logic and philosophical systems.)

Another account of jñāna-niṣṭhā practice has been given in the extracts from the end of Chapter XII of the Gītā. It refers continually to devotion to the Lord. The devotion here is not to a Lord separate from Self; it is the fourth kind of devotion, called in the Gītā 'supreme devotion', which is worship of the Lord as the Self. The key Upaniṣadic phrase, so often quoted by Śaṅkara as the core of the teachings, is: 'As the Self alone one should worship him.' He is said to be within as well as without, though words are beginning to cease to apply. The Gītā passage begins:

> XII.13 He who hates none, but is friendly and compassionate to all;
> Free from selfishness and I-ness, indifferent to pain and pleasure, patient,
>
> 14 That yogin who is always content, who is firmly self-controlled,
> Whose mind and intellect are fixed on Me in devotion, he is dear to Me.
>
> 15 Before whom the world does not tremble, and who does not tremble before the world;
> Free from thrill, haste, fear and fever, he is dear to Me.
>
> 16 Unconcerned, pure, capable, indifferent, undisturbed,
> Abandoning all undertakings, in devotion to Me, he is dear to Me.

Freedom

The Gītā has presented the supreme Self as unthinkable, but directly experienced. It has been hinted at as the end of all grief, fear, and delusion, and positively as the bliss of Brahman. When the word Brahman, absolute Reality, first comes in the Gītā, Śaṅkara defines it by three Upaniṣadic texts, one of which is: 'Brahman is consciousness-bliss.'

As Śaṅkara points out, reality cannot be accurately defined in words which are based on illusion. The most they can do is to indicate the direction of search. The search is not for something altogether unknown. If anyone can sit still for a time, throw away desires and fears, and look steadily at the mind itself and then beyond the mind, he will find there is something in him that wants to be a god.

Freedom is not the same as the idea of freedom. Take the case of people who have been imprisoned under a harsh regime for a year, through no fault of their own. Very suddenly, through the fortunes of war, they are set free in a neutral country. Imagine a husband and wife who did not expect to see each other again, and a friend who has taken some risks to help them during the captivity. The morning after release, they go for a walk on the edge of the quiet town, with its friendly people. They come to a cross-roads. 'Shall we go to the right?' says one. 'Yes, to the right, to the right.' But when they have gone a few yards, another one says, 'We could have gone straight on, couldn't we? We're free now to choose.' They burst out laughing, go back to the cross-roads and then straight on a few yards. Again they stop, look at each other, and she says solemnly, 'And what about the left one?' By now they are laughing uncontrollably: 'Yes, the left one.' And then: 'Let's sit down on the grass!' 'Let's stand up!' Everything is enjoyable, everything is comical, everything is happy. They are drunk on the idea of freedom. The fact of freedom is not affected by their laughter, but their minds are intensely aware of it, and this can go on for a time.

There are others who are equally free, but cannot free themselves from the memory of imprisonment. They are not necessarily the ones who have had objectively worse experiences; they have been more deeply affected. They look around and know they are free, but if they talk together they begin to become tense and apprehensive. Their friends try to keep them apart, and talk only about the new life. But some of them when they sleep have nightmares in which they are back in a worse prison, that of their imagination. Sometimes their friends make up a rota to sit in a comer of the bedroom with a small lamp and a book. If the sufferer begins to moan or sweat in sleep, the friend gently wakes him: 'It's all right, it's all right. You're with friends now. I'll make us a coffee and we can talk for a bit about what we're going to do tomorrow.' Again the fact of freedom is not affected by the forgetfulness of it; but the latter too can go on for a time.

When Yoga is completed, ideas drop away, even the idea 'I am Brahman'. There remains Brahman alone, the supreme Self, who as his sport projects and withdraws the seeming universes.

Free-in-Life

Release, liberation, freedom, are English words corresponding to the Sanskrit mokṣa. It means that the Self, which had been apparently confined in restrictions of a particular body-mind, shines in its own glory, the majesty of Brahman.

The seeming individual reaches the absolute freedom called mokṣa by the Path of Knowledge. As we have seen, the Knowledge when it first rises may be disturbed by memories of past associations, so vivid that they seem real. They are dissolved by jñāna-niṣṭhā, throwing away such illusions. When they have gone, the Knowledge is called by Śaṅkara 'mature', namely free from associations. Then Self remains, standing forth in its true nature, Brahman free from all associations.

Brahman, the Self, also manifests from time to time his creative power, projecting divine illusion. He enters the illusion as individual selves, accepting limitations by a conscious suspension of power and knowledge, and then struggles out of the restrictions. It is tentatively conjectured to be a joyful form of sport.

As part of the process, the Lord manifests himself as what is called Avatāra or Descent, where he takes on a divine body in order to teach himself in the human bodies. The teaching is in great part by example, and the divine body takes on many limitations. If it did not, the human beings could not take it as an example, and would be discouraged. Kṛṣṇa took on humiliation at the hands of Śiśupāla, Rāma allowed himself to be the victim of a plot to exile him for fourteen years, Jesus allowed himself to be arrested and killed. They displayed inner serenity and forgiveness, as an example. None of these sufferings was the result of past karma: the Lord has no past karma.

There is another form, which also might be called avatāra, but which Śaṅkara terms liberated-in-life. After a human being has first by karma-yoga broken free of domination by his past karma, and then by Knowledge-yoga freed himself from disturbances by memories of past karma, he is one with the Lord. The Lord is there: no one else. The Lord may take up the remaining body-mind complex and act directly as a teacher. Here he manifests feelings and intellect and will and actions, but without disturbance of the inner serenity of the Self. The difference from the jñāna-niṣṭhā stage of the Path of Knowledge is that in jñāna-niṣṭhā the movements of mind are spontaneous and may temporarily disturb, whereas in the Liberated-in-life, they are consciously taken up, and do not disturb. One on the Path of Knowledge can be compared to one released from prison, who knows he is free but occasionally is attacked by a feeling of being still held. It is best for him to keep away from the sight of prisons for a time. The liberated-in-life corresponds to an ex-prisoner who is now a prison visitor to the prison camp. He is in the prison with the others, eats the same food and so on. But he is not oppressed by it. He enjoys doing all that can be done to help the prisoners towards remission of their sentence by good conduct.

It is asked: How can teaching be undertaken at all, by one who 'sees the Self in all, and all in the Self'? What could it possibly mean? There is no one else for him to teach.

In answer, it has to be said again that we cannot expect to describe realization of unity in terms of words, which are based on separateness. But a seer gave an answer in six words: The whole world is his body.

The analogy may satisfy the mind enough to allow practice. A pianist, like most people, regards the body as himself. He trains the fingers assiduously, recognizing the defects in movement and precision. At those times, he treats the fingers as other than himself. He imposes exercises on them, but he does not curse them for clumsiness. All pianists have to give special training to the fourth and fifth fingers, because they are only partially independent of each other. The virtuoso pianist Robert Schumann, an occasionally unstable genius, began to hate these fingers for their relative inefficiency. He tried to remedy it by forcible physical means, and destroyed himself as a performer. (He met the disaster courageously, however, by going in for composition.)

Those who have done any training in physical skills like typing, or in mental fields like logic or memory, recognize the situation. While being trained, the body, or mind, is something other. Its weaknesses have to be seen clearly, and patiently corrected. But outside the training period, it is oneself. On the deepest level, of course, it is always the Self. This is one analogy for teaching by the liberated-while-living.

What of the Hitlers and Stalins, who were worshipped by so many? Most of us, looking calmly and carefully, will recognize times when we ourselves have worshipped some Hitler or Stalin in ourselves. Only later does realization come of the harm that has been done. Not many of us do well when suddenly in a position of power.

If it is not stretching the analogy too far, perhaps the Liberated-in-life sees the actual Hitler and Stalin in the Self, and the Self in the Hitler and Stalin. They have to be opposed, but they are not outside the Self. They must have done some good in the past to be elevated to power; then they had choice, and they turned their faces downward. After long sufferings, they will again come to the opportunity to make a choice. Perhaps then, the deep latent impression of the past failure will help to turn their faces upward. One teacher used to say: 'We have all been Nero, we have all been Judas, we have all been Hulagu who burnt Baghdad and many of its citizens alive. Now we have choice again. What will we decide to be now?'

The Liberated-in-life stands before us, saying: 'Will you not walk with me this time?'

PART IV

Pointers for Practice

The Experimental Basis

XIII.24 By meditation, some see the Self in the self by the self.

VI.27 Supreme bliss comes to the yogin who is pure, passion laid to rest, his mind stilled; he becomes Brahman.

The Gītā is a textbook of yoga (a word which has also the sense of 'method' and 'addition'). It is not an intellectual or religious analysis ending up in blind belief or disbelief.

The ancient Bṛhadāraṇyaka Upaniṣad of at least 600 BC declared: 'To this day whoever thus knows It as "I am Brahman" becomes universal.' Śaṅkara, over a thousand years later, commented: 'Some might think that they were gods in those days with wonderful powers, whereas the weak mortals of today could never do it. But that is not so. Brahman is the Self of all beings, and their apparent differences in power are illusory.' Over a thousand years later still, Dr Shastri gave the same assurance: 'Through the holy yoga, anyone who is one-pointedly determined will attain God-realization.'

Some modern readers do not understand the force of an experimental tradition. They say there are contradictions in the Gītā, and central concepts which merely reflect ideas of the day. So an ancient text like this should be sifted critically, rejecting, for instance, the contradictions, but retaining at least provisionally what we think has value for modern conditions. Such critics suffer from a fallacy, not so much logical as psychological, which can be called the Fallacy of Fluctuating Premises. They base their criticisms of yoga on premises which they do not, and cannot, accept when examining their present-day conclusions. The Fallacy can be illustrated from the history of the theory of light.

Newton in the eighteenth century suggested that light was a stream of corpuscles; Thomas Young at the beginning of the nineteenth century demonstrated the phenomenon of diffraction, which seemed to establish an old wave theory, which had lost out to Newton. There was a heated debate: Young was even accused of lack of patriotism in opposing Newton's theory The corpuscular school and the wave school were totally opposed. In his great mid-century works like *The History of the Inductive Sciences*, William Whewell pointed out that the wave theory could explain problems not even thought of when it was first proposed, whereas the corpuscular theory had to be repeatedly adapted to meet new evidence. This, he remarked, is a great test of the validity of a theory. He admitted that some English scientists (he had just invented the word), working with very weak sources of light, were still opposed. But there was no doubt (he concluded) that the difficulties they pointed out would be due simply to incidental experimental error, and all the younger men would accept the wave theory.

This indeed happened: the wave theory held the field till the beginning of the twentieth century. Then came the discovery of the photoelectric effect (working also with very weak sources of light), and its Nobel Prize-winning explanation by Einstein. Light was now analysed as a stream of particles – photons. But diffraction could not be denied. Light had a dual nature: wave-like and particle-like. Numerous other experiments extended this to electron beams, and even neutron beams. A fundamental anomaly appeared at the heart of physics: with waves of like nature, when a peak meets a trough they can annihilate each other, but not so with like particles.

It is a contradiction, as Einstein repeatedly calls it in his book *The Evolution of Physics*. But experiments do not contradict each other: it is ideas about them which contradict. These last are often based on unconscious extension of childhood experiences, with, for instance, seawaves and pebbles. We have to be prepared to give up nineteenth-century mechanistic deterministic preconceptions.

The experiments in yoga are performed and repeated: they are accepted as they stand. They are not to be criticized on the basis of nineteenth-century concepts, supposedly modem and scientific, but in fact long ago discarded.

Yoga has the advantage that it can be practised, and confirmed, in nearly every human life: it is not a question of reading about proceedings in distant laboratories.

A second common occasion of the Fallacy of Fluctuating Premises comes in regard to reported experiences in yoga. The Mephistopheles in most people takes a text like Gītā XIII.32, which refers to the Self as space-like. He thumps his fist on the table, looks at it, and says: 'Rather difficult to imagine this as space, isn't it?'

Here is an artist's impression of the atoms on the point of a needle. The doubter may be asked: 'Do you believe your body consists of atoms?'

'Certainly. Science tells us that.'

'And you accept that the nucleus, in relation to the whole atom, is about the dimensions of a walnut in a football field? The rest is space. You agree?'

'Yes, I suppose so. They do say that.'

'But do you actually believe, sitting here at the table, that your fist and whole body, and the table, are almost entirely space?'

'To that, I can reply unhesitatingly ... Ye – e – s.'

This typical little exchange – often wholly internal – shows the Fallacy of Fluctuating Premises. The premise of naive realism (in this case identification with the body-image), is adopted in order to rule out yoga, but cannot be maintained as science, which in fact refutes it. As Russell said, in a remark admired by Einstein: 'Naive realism, if true, is false; therefore it is false.'

Yoga is based on direct empirical and then transcendental experience, which can be only roughly indicated in words and concepts derived from the present life of restriction and illusion.

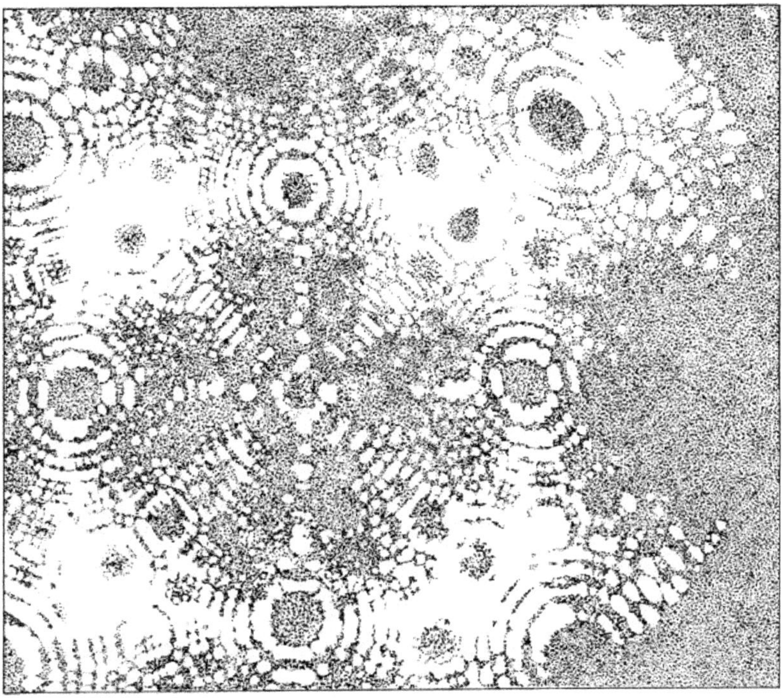

Atoms on the point of a needle

Artist's impression of atoms on the point of a needle. They are 'silhouetted' as the dark round spots against a stream of ions in a vacuum. At the centre of each atom is the nucleus, the only thing that could be called matter. If the atom were the size of a football pitch, the nucleus would be walnut-sized. (Could the much-ridiculed Scholastic debate, on angels dancing on a needlepoint, have been a guess at the possibility of higher dimensions?)

Mistakes

A pupil who lived rather carelessly remarked: 'Mistakes are a necessary part of the path of training. If you read the biographies of even the greatest, they all say that they made many mistakes. Some of them say that mistakes are necessary – one learns from them. So I don't worry about my own conduct: let the mistakes come, I think, let 'em all come. I'll go through them and come out the other side. It is all part of the path.'

This was put to a senior pupil, a business woman, for her opinion. She remarked: 'You need not tell him I said this, but I don't think our teacher would rate the idea very high in terms of clear thinking. It's easy to get woolly about spiritual things. I remember when I learnt to type. It was in a class. Of course we made mistakes, but the teacher always stressed the importance of getting the habit of absolutely accurate typing. He never said that as mistakes are inevitable in learning to type, let 'em all come. He told us we should type very slowly, if necessary, to reduce the mistakes to almost nil. Those of us who followed his advice finally learnt to type with perfect accuracy without thinking about it.

The others, though at first they typed a bit quicker, were always subject to occasional lapses and never became good typists.

'Mistakes are like the falls when one is taking up skating. Some are inevitable, but we should make them as few as possible. They are part of the path, it is true, but they are stumbles, not forward steps.'

The Well

Some students discourage themselves by looking at themselves each day. After trying hard for a session, they feel that as there has been no result they have failed. Next day they try again, and again they fail. Gradually this builds up into a conviction of continuous failure, and they begin to think: 'Oh, what's the use of trying?'

For such occasions there is an ancient Indian example, that of the well-digger. The Indian tradition was that beneath the desert there is water, however deeply hidden. (This has recently been confirmed in the case of the vast Rajasthan desert in north-west India, beneath which a legendary river was supposed to flow. It has been established that the river is actually there, though deep underground.) The maxim of the well-digger is this. Each day when he digs but finds no water, he does not think: 'I have failed.' Next day he digs again, deeper, and so on day after day. Every evening, though he has found no water yet, he thinks not, 'I have failed,' but, 'Nearer, nearer, nearer!'

The Four Vocations

IV.13 The four-class system was created by Me
In accordance with distinctions of guṇa-s and results-of-actions (karma).

XVIII.41–4 The actions of Brahmins, of warriors, of businessmen, and of those who do service,
Are distinguished according to the guṇa-s that come up out of their inborn nature.

Calm, self-control, austerity (tapas), purity, patience and uprightness,
Knowledge theoretical and practical, faith – are the nature-born behaviour of the Brahmin.

Heroism, majesty, firmness, resourcefulness, not yielding in fight,
Generosity, dignity – are the nature-born behaviour of the warrior.

> Farming and trade are the nature-born behaviour of businessmen;
>
> Service is the nature-born vocation of those who are drawn to it.

The Laws of Manu lay down general rules that a Brahmin, for instance, should be the son or daughter of two Brahmin parents. However this represents a hardening into a fixed social rule of what is merely a natural tendency – that the son of a carpenter (a much more important profession then than now) will probably develop an aptitude for building, or the son of a scholar, for scholarship. Manu himself recognizes in places the defects of a fixed rule of heredity; he says in II.87: 'he who befriends all creatures is declared to be a Brahmin', and elsewhere: 'a Brahmin who lacks piety and learning, and an elephant made of leather – there is nothing there but the name.'

In the oldest spiritual classics the divisions were not made automatically on the basis of heredity, as they later tended to be. In the Chāndogya Upaniṣad, one of the oldest, a would-be pupil who is illegitimate, is asked by the teacher about his parentage. He answers: 'Sir, I am illegitimate; and I know only my mother's name.' The teacher says at once: 'I will take you as a pupil. Only a true Brahmin would thus fearlessly speak out the truth.' This shows that the determinant of spiritual class was the inner character, not parentage.

The Gītā several times refers to the four classes: Brahmin, warrior, businessman, and server. It nowhere says that they are determined by parentage; rather it is by their inborn tendencies, which have however to be cultivated. They correspond to what today we should call a vocation. As the Gītā says, the vocation may be missed: 'the vocation of another brings on anxiety.'

The Gītā speaks of the duties (not of any rights) which a given role entails. The Brahmin, for instance, was to be non-violent, but he had to speak out the truth fearlessly regardless of consequences to himself. There are striking illustrations of this in early Upaniṣads, where the Brahmin has fallen away from his vocation and become a ritualist, with only a theoretical knowledge of the Self. In some of these passages, it is a king who teaches the Brahmin the kingly secret of yogic action, on a far higher plane than rituals. One element in the Brahmin's role was to be a transmitter of these sacred texts, and it is a tribute to their integrity that they faithfully preserved even such sections where the Brahmin comes off second-best to the king. The Gītā, given by a warrior to a warrior, is in the same tradition of the kingly secret. There is a notable example in Chapter X, when the Lord is teaching that He is to be seen as the best of each class of things: 'Of men, I am the king' (X.27).

A great temptation for the warrior was power, whereas the businessman was regarded as specially in danger of selfishness. But the Gītā emphasizes that if they pursue their occupation faithfully as an offering to the Lord, in serenity of mind, they attain the same inner purity and clarity as any Brahmin. And so too with the role of service. They all qualify for Knowledge and the Knowledge path, as Śaṅkara states unambiguously in his commentary to XVIII.46.

When the system hardened into hereditary succession, the servers or śūdra class finally became desperately downtrodden. But this was not the intention. There are many who do not feel equal to facing the changes of fortune by their own power. They wish to join some group which they respect, and serve it without having to take much responsibility for decisions. They can do immense good with their unselfish service to some admired reforming movement, though not understanding everything about it. Leaders who begin to look with contempt on such faithful followers undermine, and finally destroy, their own movement.

In fact, the Gītā presentation of all four classes is in terms of service: duties, not rights. The Brahmin served Truth, and served others with truth; the warrior served with organization, and protection of the weak; the businessman served by creating wealth for the community; the servers served directly, as members of a group.

The key to the Gītā allocation of vocations is given in the next two verses:

> XVIII.45 Taking delight in his own special role, the human being attains perfection:
> Listen now to how it is reached, by one delighting in his own special role:
>
> 46 One attains perfection by worshipping the Lord with his own appropriate action,
> The Lord from whom comes all action, and by whom all this is pervaded.

The word 'delight' shows that the role proper to that person is one which will give inner fulfilment; it is not a question of duty done, a pledge honoured, an undertaking doggedly carried through. There is to be a delight in it, attesting that it is creative. Dr Shastri used to tell his pupils that there is for everyone a particular way in which he or she can serve in worship, and that such service when discovered and performed gives a deep inner satisfaction. It arises from the Lord who is the Self. It is not a matter of having been born in a particular 'caste'. Dr Shastri himself was born in a Brahmin family, with a lineage going back to Upaniṣadic sages. But he followed his father in giving up Brahminical privileges and distinctions as they were then claimed in India. 'One who seeks for Brahman is a Brahmin,' he used to quote to his students.

At the beginning of the Gītā, Arjuna laments hysterically the disastrous effects of war on family and class lineage, and says he will not be guilty of such a sin. But it is clear that all this is merely an excuse for getting out of what he does not want to do. If these were his true convictions, he would have thought of them before, instead of boasting of what he was going to do in the battle. As a matter of fact, at the time of the events related by the Gītā, there was not this rigid idea of class distinction by birth. The matter can be tested by looking at a few of the most prominent figures in the Gītā.

Vyāsa (the word is a title meaning 'compiler '), who arranged the Vedas, might be expected to be a pillar of orthodox descent. But he was illegitimate, offspring of a casual amour. His mother Satyavatī, later a famous queen, went to an islet in the river to bear him, and named him simply Kānīna (Bastard). He was subsequently called Kṛṣṇa, 'dark' (from his dark colour), and Dvaipāyana or 'island-born'. Satyavatī married a king, by whom she had two sons, both of whom died childless. The king also died. As with other early societies, in which many children died, in such a case a brother could be asked to deputize for a dead husband. Vyāsa was only half-brother, and himself illegitimate; however he acceded to Satyavatī's request. The king had left two widows, who gave birth respectively to Dhṛtarāṣṭra, born blind but later the king, and Pāṇḍu. The five Pāṇḍava heroes take their patronymic from him (Pāṇḍu: Pāṇḍava). But here again they were not his sons, but only adopted. Pāṇḍu's wife Kuntī had received the boon of being visited by six gods, by whom she had six children: Yudhiṣṭhira, Arjuna, Bhīma, two twins who do not figure in the Gītā, and Karṇa whom she abandoned. He was found and adopted by a charioteer. So all the Pāṇḍavas were also illegitimate, including Arjuna. That was doubtless why he was so sensitive on the point, repeatedly sneering at Karṇa as 'that son of a charioteer' (Gītā XI.26).

Of other great characters referred to in the Gītā, Bhīṣma was only half human, one parent being the spirit of the Ganges. Droṇa did not have a mother at all; nevertheless he counted as a Brahmin, and his killer paid the penalty of slaying a Brahmin.

Thus the main characters of the Gītā itself were of irregular parentage. Some of the accounts may well be symbolic, but their acceptance shows that in the Gītā view the so-called caste distinctions were not at all rigid. Caste is from the Portuguese, the original Sanskrit word being varṇa, literally colour. It has been proposed that there was an intention of distinguishing the later invaders, fairer-skinned Aryans, from the earlier invaders, the dark-skinned Dravidians. However, as noted above, one name for Vyāsa, arranger of the Veda, the sacred scriptures of the Aryans, was Kṛṣṇa, meaning dark, blue-black, or black. It is also the name of the avatāra or divine descent who gives the Gītā itself. He is dark. It is his brother, Balarāma, who is fair-skinned.

The conclusion is that in the Gītā the distinctions are based on inner vocation. The proper role in life is literally a 'calling', and not an accident of birth. But there is the likelihood that in many cases the circumstances of a family profession or trade would tend to bring out any latent tendencies in the same direction. Śaṅkara points out that when the highest calling comes, the calling to Self-realization, it supersedes the seemingly absolute claims of worldly roles, and the Gītā says to the advanced pupil:

> XVIII.66 Giving up all duties, turn to Me alone.
> I will free you from all difficulties: do not grieve.

Uprush

Yogic action begins with following the traditional instructions on life, but it cannot remain a question of obedience, sometimes cheerful and sometimes reluctant. There might be no time to think, 'What ought I to do?' If yoga has been practised faithfully, habits of right action are set up which cover most cases. But the time comes when things are not clear: perhaps duties conflict, or cause suffering to innocent people.

The yoga practices of meditation lay down luminous, semi-transparent saṃskāra-impressions at the root of the mind. At first these are mostly just good thinking-patterns and good action-patterns, which reproduce what has been contemplated on. But as the translucent areas become wider, shafts of light begin to shine through them. Then there are inspirations which have nothing to do with limitation.

Suppose it is necessary to take a considerable risk for a good cause. The yogin's first feeling may be to try to escape, but then he screws his resolution up to it. This is a great victory in a yogic career. What has been practised at special times, in safety, is now brought to life in the middle of danger. Yet there is something higher still. When he has practised earnestly – not necessarily for a very long time, but earnestly – and the situation is put to him, he feels to his surprise an uprush in his spirit: 'Yes, yes, come on, come on!' A normally rather timid person is amazed at the daring coming from the unknown depths.

There can be agonizing decisions to be taken, both alternatives of which are equally unthinkable. (This is the Gītā situation, at the beginning.) A foreign student on a visit to a dictatorship gets to know one of the local students. The foreign student sometimes talks about politics. Without telling anyone, he smuggles in some officially unwelcome literature and leaves it in public places. The police find copies, and begin an inquiry. The foreign student is advised by his embassy (who have a good idea what has happened) to leave the country; they will get him out quickly. He is about to agree, when he hears in a roundabout way that the police are thinking of pinning the offence on to his friend, who knows nothing about it.

He tells the embassy that if the friend is arrested, he will himself go and own up. The wise old embassy Counsellor tells him privately: It would do no good at all; they'd simply sentence both of you. I've been in this country thirty years, and I know. The police don't like him, and they never let anyone go that they don't like. Go home – you can't do anything by staying.'

What is he to do? He can go, but if his friend is arrested, he may be plagued by guilt all his life. After all, the Counsellor might be wrong; having got the real culprit, the police might find it awkward to arrest someone else as well. But if he stays on, every morning he will have the apprehensive thought: 'Will it be today?'

In the case of a yogin, something completely different rises which frees him from both alternatives. No one who has not been through this sort of experience has the right to suggest particular 'solutions'; in any case people do not believe them.

Here are some comments on the general principle given by Dr Shastri in his book A *Path to God-realization*, published in China for the Chinese public as well as his own pupils.

> Life has proved to me that at times the mind also becomes helpless and confused and cannot then be relied upon. The mind says, 'All is over', but at such moments a light superior to the mind flashes within and guides my thoughts, which were submerged in hopelessness, to quite unanticipated regions. In the twinkling of an eye all sorrow vanishes, problems are solved, the knot of fate is untied.
>
> Be it remembered that the human mind never recommends to itself self-sacrifice or absolute self-abnegation. The power which produces these conditions must, therefore, be beyond the mind.
>
> Whence does the inspiration come? This superior power is the light of Ātman, the spirit of man, flashing through the psychic medium called the heart.
>
> > Gītā XV. 19 He who, undeluded, knows the supreme Spirit, knows all....
>
> (Śaṇkara's comment: by becoming the Spirit which is the Self of all things, he knows them ... this is what is meant by saying that he knows all.)

It is natural to ask: What can these old texts on yoga give to me in my present life? And anyway, how do I know that they are true?

One of the features of yoga practice is that there are small confirmations almost from the very beginning. They can come even to people who are not formally practising it at all. To study yoga theory can make us aware of spiritual events in daily life which otherwise just get overlooked. Or else people say: 'Wasn't that extraordinary!' but then shift it onto a sort of mental siding, because it doesn't seem to fit in with ordinary experience.

So, long before a great realization like that of the verse 'He who undeluded knows the supreme Spirit ...' these can be small inspirations; they can happen to anyone whose mind is relatively calm, and unselfishly concentrated on a good end. In fact, inspirations are raining on to all minds from the supreme Spirit all the time, but those who are darkened and agitated by selfish passions cannot understand them.

We see the same thing when we begin to study science.

When our eyes are opened to the laws of physics, for example, we begin to realize that these laws are operating everywhere and all the time. But we will see the operation clearly only when the circumstances are favourable. For instance, it is very difficult to see gravity working on leaves in a hurricane. They are carried high into the air; though gravity is pulling all the time, its effect is masked and apparently reversed by the action of the wind. In the same way, the effect of divine inspiration is masked and apparently contradicted by the gale of selfish passion.

On a calm day in autumn, the action of gravity on falling leaves is more clearly seen, though still a bit distorted by wind resistance. It was perfectly shown only in the vacuum on the moon surface, when the astronaut was filmed dropping a piece of lead and a feather side by side, and they reached the surface together. Similarly, in a calm and clear mind, the action of inspiration from the supreme Spirit is clearer, though it becomes perfectly received only in the complete stillness of samādhi meditation.

Examples of inspiration in worldly life are often given (in the West) from the lives of great scientists, or (in the East) from those of great artists. Many of them are very convincing, because they are well attested. They were so famous that their inspirations were recorded. The disadvantage is, that we may come to think inspiration must be associated with technical mastery of some specialized field.

It can be somehow frustrating to hear about inspirations of scientists and artists, and then be told that this same inspiration can transform our own everyday life. We need examples of it in people not gifted with great talents. But the difficulty is, that now there is no evidence in support; no one has heard of these people and it all seems just stories.

Still, there are cases where the solutions speak for themselves. Sometimes it is the application of a traditional saying, such as the Zen one about Shutting the Door. Dr Shastri (who had lived and taught for years in Japan and China) once quoted it for his pupils.

> In an old-style Japanese hotel, a guest has his own room, and the maid brings the meals there. One day, over-worked and tired, she doesn't close the door fully when she goes out.
>
> If the guest is an inconsiderate man who does not notice the girl's fatigue and simply demands value for his money, he shouts: 'Oi! Shut that door!'
>
> If it is a scholar, he calls politely: 'Shut the door, would you please?'
>
> But if it is a man of Zen, he gets up and shuts it himself.

Often after hearing such a story, we think, 'How beautiful,' and pass on to something else. But it is meant to be applied in life. How can it be applied? one wonders; we do not have the situation here.

But take the case of an ambitious teenager studying for examinations. His teachers say that if he studies at home five evenings a week for a year, he can get the necessary grades. He wants to do it, but finds it harder and harder to settle down to his books in the evening in his bedroom while the parents are watching television. They keep it low, but he knows it is on. He begins to stay to watch a bit himself, and this bit gets longer and longer. Now perhaps the father has a row with him: 'You've taken this on, and you'll damned well go through with it, like I had to at your age. Or I won't lift a finger to help you get started in life afterwards.' This may have some effect, but it can also produce lifelong resentment. The mother may try gentle persuasion: 'It's only for a year – tell yourself that. It's only a year. I'll bring you some coffee and a sandwich at nine o'clock, dear. Anything you want, you just tell me. You know we all want to help.' Again it may have some effect, but that effect soon wears off. Then what to do?

Suppose the parents have practised a spiritual path, and heard something like the Zen Shut the Door! story How is it to be applied? They meditate on it, and there is an inspiration. Father ponders, 'There's that diploma I've often thought of going in for. It's not directly in my line, but it would be quite an advantage to have it. It'd take about a year.' And mother has an idea too: 'I've always wanted to try embroidery; I could find an evening class round here, and go once a week, and do it at home the other week-days.'

So without any fuss, a new routine begins on week-day evenings. When the table is cleared after the early evening meal, the television is shut down, father gets out some books and paper, and mother gets out her sewing. The son now finds it easy to study: everyone is studying.

The father's shout, 'You'll damned well do it!' – that was the shout of Shut the Door! The mother's plea, 'It's only a year, dear' – that was the Please Shut the Door. But when they themselves began studying – that was shutting the door oneself.

One could think: 'Well, that is after all an idea that could come to almost anyone; it is true that most people don't seem to think of it, but still, I wouldn't have to call it inspiration.' There is a much clearer instance in what Dr Watson would have called The Curious Affair of the State Coach.

By the nineteenth century, the British Coronation ritual was the most ancient in Europe; but in practice it was nothing like the much rehearsed and brilliantly stage-managed ceremonials of today. Reigns were often short; the Earl Marshal, traditionally in charge, would in his lifetime normally see about three such ceremonies: first as a junior helping his father, then in charge himself, and finally as an adviser in the background. There were records of the outline of the ceremonies, but the details were from memory: Do what was done last time.

However when Edward VII finally came to the throne, and was to be crowned in 1902, there was a difficulty. His mother Queen Victoria had become Queen as a young girl in 1837, and there was no one still living who had had anything to do with the coronation arrangements. The Earl Marshal, the Duke of Norfolk, was a mild-mannered and conscientious man, though not (by all accounts) over-burdened with brains. He and his committee determined that everything should go perfectly. To forestall any untoward happenings, they would follow exactly the coronation ceremony of the young Queen Victoria. They had to shuffle through a great deal of paper to find out details. He wrote in his diary that he thought of it day and night. They got a little more time when the King suddenly fell ill, and had to be operated on for appendicitis. Finally everything was settled. There was no time for a full-scale rehearsal, but the main characters in the ritual knew their parts – though with some anxious moments in the case of the octogenarian Archbishop of Canterbury. (In the event, the King had to hold him up at one point.)

The Earl Marshal noted in his diary that at last he felt that they had completed their task. He put away the papers, dismissed his secretary, and went to bed. He slept briefly, but then found himself awake, with the feeling that there was something wrong. He tried to brush it aside: they had all gone over the whole thing again and again. There was no possible mistake, none. But he could not sleep.

When he realized that he was going to be awake, he took a decision that shows considerable character. He may not have been too bright intellectually, but he could think constructively. Instead of mindlessly worrying over something that he could not specify, he resolved to pass the time by calmly picturing in full detail the whole event, just as they had planned it. He had been thinking of it continuously, and in the quiet of the bedroom, yet wide awake, he would easily have passed into a state of complete concentration.

He saw himself turning up at Buckingham Palace in very good time; there was no worry that the King would not be ready, but he had to check with one of the ladies-in-waiting that the Queen's distressing tendency to lateness was under control. Punctually at eleven o'clock the royal pair got into the golden state coach, built by Sir W. Chambers in 1760 at a cost of £8,000, and which had carried the young Queen Victoria to Westminster Abbey for her own coronation sixty-four years before. The coach is enclosed, and has a sort of ornamental top-knot on its roof. Behind an escort of cuirassiers, the eight cream-coloured horses began to pull the coach; he watched with satisfaction its dignified pace along the Mall.

Following the route taken by Queen Victoria, the carriage turned right before the great Admiralty Arch, and went across the open parade ground towards the much smaller arch of the Horse Guards. It would pass under that arch into Whitehall. The Earl Marshal surveyed its progress in his mind's eye.

It was just entering the darkness of the arch ... now it would come out. ... But no, it did not. He made the picture again. It would go through the arch, and come out. ... But he could not get the carriage through. He knew that this very state coach, with the young Queen Victoria in it, had gone through that very arch. Yet now – for some reason – it would not. There could be no reason, but – he could not get the state coach through the arch.

As soon as it was light, he sent an urgent message to his secretary to come at once, with a carpenter's rule and tape measure. They went first to the stables, and carefully measured the height of the top of the state coach. Then they went to the Horse Guards arch, and measured its maximum height. Two inches too low: the coach would not go through.

Hastily the route was re-planned, and the state coach went instead under the huge Admiralty Arch, to turn right into Whitehall, as it does on State occasions today.

The diary does not speculate on possible explanations: perhaps the ground under the arch had been repaired and raised a little, or perhaps the arch had sunk a little in sixty years, or perhaps in the refurbishment of the state coach, the wheel-rims had been replaced by thicker ones.

The important point is that it was an inspiration, a 'truth-bearing knowledge' in the words of Patañjali, who says that this comes to one who had practised pure single-minded concentration on a particular thing for a good time. The inspiration was against the logic of the situation, though with hindsight we can see that it was not illogical. Logical thinking might suggest: 'Check on the remote chance that the relative heights of the coach and arch might have changed.' However the inspiration was not like that. It did not say: 'Check!' but gave the result before any check had been made.

A second point to notice is that it was not one of those vague premonitions of a distracted mind, noticed when they come true but forgotten or discounted ('well, I wasn't really sure, you know') when they do not. True inspiration comes to a mind that has concentrated unselfishly and one-pointedly for a considerable time on the same thing, and when it finally enters a state of quiet meditation.

One may ask: why don't these things happen more often? As a rule, they come once and then no more. One reason is, that the surprising success usually arouses selfishness in the mind. Then the conditions for inspiration are disturbed. The feeling comes: 'I've done it once, and I can do it again. I can really make something out of this.' It is quite difficult to rise above the excitement and anticipation. The experience of the sages who were experts in yoga is that without regular and earnest meditation practice it can hardly be done. When selfish illusions rise, they are like a cloud of smoke, cutting us off from the sunshine of inspiration, and this is why the Gītā verse quoted at the beginning said: 'undeluded'. The mind-sky must be clear.

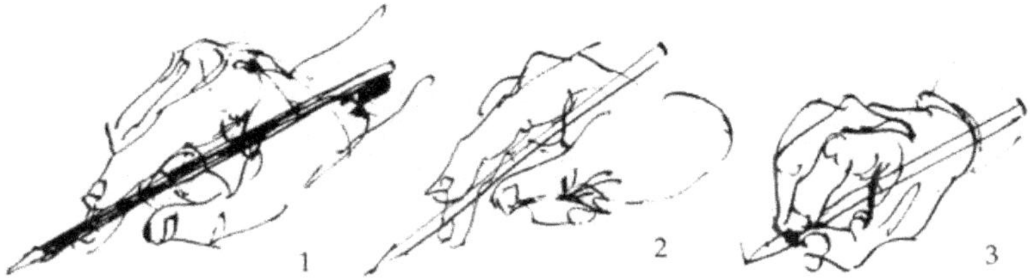

Writing: Love, no Love

1 The nature of the pencil is long. So it should be held well down the shaft, balanced by middle and index fingers, with thumb coming on afterwards to help steer.
2 When control has been learnt, the pencil can cover a wide sweep, and the hand does not have to be continually moved. High-speed shorthand reporters, holding in this way, can write a whole line with perfect precision, without needing to move the hand. Once mastered, it is natural and easy.
3 The pencil is held as if it were a stub, tightly pinched between finger-tips and a bent thumb. It is treated as an enemy, and often there is much needless pressure. The hand has to be moved for each word, and it is unnatural and tiring.

Human Nature

> III.33 People act in conformity with their own nature – even the wise man;
> Beings follow their nature: what can forcible restraint avail?

'It's only human nature' is an excuse often made. It rests on the unspoken assumption that human nature is unchangeable – an eternally boiling spring of desire, anger and other passions, which can be held down for a time, but must then burst out with redoubled force, perhaps in concealed form.

The Gītā analysis is quite different. Human nature is the latent deposit of dynamic seeds laid down previously; they include impulses to balance, peace and goodwill to all. If these last are encouraged, the seed-bed changes, and the impulses from it become lucid, well directed and calm.

At the deepest level of all, approachable through yoga practice, there is a drive to be free from all restrictions. On the superficial levels, the restrictions are most immediately felt as anger, sex-desire, and greed:

> XVI.21 Threefold is the hell-gate leading to self- destruction:
> The three are pleasure-craving, wrath, and greed, and they
> must be given up.

They must be given up because they become compulsive, blindly repetitive in the one whom they possess, regardless of the circumstances. Anger, which first had an object, becomes free-ranging; the slightest check or surprise, almost anything, makes him angry. The man of desire no longer enjoys the object: he simply cannot do without it. The man of greed accumulates more and more things out of habit; he has forgotten why he wanted them in the first place.

Anger should be looked at first, because it most directly harms others. Moreover, today it is realized that it is possible to control anger, and even dispel it, by a conscious attempt to recognize the common humanity in the other party.

It is understood that tribal or clan enmities, though 'natural' and found everywhere, can be changed into something like a cultural or sporting rivalry which leads not to hate but friendship. We dimly realize today that there need not always be some urge to kill buried under precarious self-control. Many countries which now feel themselves a unity once consisted of bitterly warring tribes. Others have not yet succeeded in doing this, but at least it is known to be possible. It is not ruled out on the ground that 'you cannot change human nature'.

Friends, or nurses, who have to subdue someone in delirium, or even fighting drunk, feel a flash of anger when punched in the face. But it vanishes as they recognize the noble human being behind the contorted features. That humanity is temporarily overcast, but it is there. Admittedly force has to be used, but it is minimum force, and used without hate.

The yogin looks through the events of the world. He tries to find out, in meditation, what his self as an individual is to do for the clearer and clearer manifestation of the great Self as universal. Very hostile circumstances are like tempests: he battles against them while they last, but does not waste energy hating them.

Physical pleasure has become a sort of ideal to many people. But it is a frustrating ideal because it is inherently very short, depending as it does on change. To illustrate the traditional Indian analysis, Dr Shastri told his pupils to observe how after the second mouthful, the pleasure in the food progressively lessens.

Regulation of pleasure is essential for its continuance. Chinese art teaches the lesson that space is an integral part of the picture: it is not simply a blank. Similarly restraint in enjoyment is not frustration, but an integral part of it. Without restraint, what began as pleasure becomes first mechanical and then joylessly compulsive.

The Gītā was given to Arjuna, a married man, and celibacy is not enjoined on the karma-yogin. But a rather strict control is essential, to preserve physical vigour and prevent mental enslavement and depression.

There is a view today that frequent sexual intercourse, regular or casual, is a prime necessity for health and personal fulfilment. It claims the support of Freud, but is a travesty of his view. (He held that all culture is based on repression and sublimation, and that the reality principle must control the pleasure principle.)

The idea is based on a myth, comparable to the medieval European myth of meat-eating. The nobles took four enormous meals daily, of strengthening meat, with occasional fish. Dairy products and vegetables were held to be positively weakening. We estimate today that the lower classes, if not actually starving, lived on a far healthier diet than the nobles; there is some evidence that they lived longer.

The myth that meat diet is essential for martial virtue is baseless. In the Japanese age of clan wars, conspicuous bravery, and strategy, were shown by the non-meat-eating generals and their armies up to 20,000 strong. (Compare the 15,000 English at Agincourt.)

Today, good observation and experiment have shown that good health requires very much less food in quantity, and little or even no meat.

When the unquestioned sex-myth is subjected to observation and experiment, it is likely that similar conclusions will be reached in regard to compulsive addiction.

There is another myth, again without foundation, that it is in this that man demonstrates manhood. But, as Dr Shastri remarked half-humorously, a wolf can do as much. Man, the biped, on this occasion becomes a quadruped. He demonstrates manhood in development of the higher faculties. Dr Shastri often cited Goethe as one of the high-water marks of Western civilization, and Goethe wrote:

> Let man be noble,
> for that alone sets him apart
> from the animals ...

Those who undertake a serious attempt to realize the Self have to be prepared to give up excitement, and develop the deeper pleasure of inner tranquillity and then vision.

'Aren't I allowed to enjoy my cup of tea?'

'You don't enjoy your cup of tea, because as you drink it, your head is boiling with hope of this and fear of that, and what you're going to do, and what you might have done. When your mind is clear and calm, you'll enjoy the cup of tea. And you'll enjoy just as much when it's not there.'

Greed is not rated highly nowadays as a theoretical ideal. But it is still very powerful in practice. Fundamentally it is based on a deep fear of something unknown; possessions are felt to be a protective wall. Some few things are needed for life in the world, but greed piles them up mindlessly When envy is a motive, greed is specially compulsive. As a Far Eastern proverb has it: 'Envious people are always counting the money in others' pockets.'

The Spiritual Teacher

The Bhagavad Gītā is a teaching for crisis. In many ways it is quite different from the situations in the Upaniṣads, where a seeker after truth attends on a teacher. The Upaniṣadic procedure is however described in a group of Gītā verses beginning with IV.34, in the context of Knowledge:

> Go to those who have knowledge and have realized it directly. Learn by bowing down, by questioning, and by being attentive; They will teach you Knowledge.

The word translated 'being attentive' is literally 'service', but Śaṅkara here and elsewhere explains it as basically 'wanting to hear'. It is not simply slavish obedience for its own sake.

At the beginning of the Gītā, Arjuna is not yet a disciple in these terms. He is not seeking truth: he does ask, but not about bondage and spiritual freedom, only about what he should do in this particular crisis. He does not bow down to Kṛṣṇa; he simply respects him as a friend of good judgment. Though he does say once, 'I am your disciple, tell me what to do', he goes on without reverence, calling him by familiar nicknames such as Keṣava. It means someone with a shock of hair, which might correspond to the English 'Curly'. He is later overwhelmed at the thought of how casual and irreverent he has been. He bows down then, but that is not till Chapter XI. Moreover, Arjuna has done no service to Kṛṣṇa, nor asked him questions about knowledge of truth. How is it then that the teaching of the Gītā – which proclaims itself to be Upaniṣadic – is given to him?

It is a case of what our teacher Dr Shastri called the 'dharma of emergency'. In an emergency, preconditions may be set aside. He used to give the example of a doctor. In classical times the sick person's household would send a formal invitation to the doctor (and a carriage if they could afford it). The doctor himself must dress carefully, arrange his things in good order, and proceed with dignified bearing to the place. But if it were an emergency, the doctor must drop everything else and run barefoot. So in Arjuna's case, the requirements are waived, even the inner requirements of full faith in the spiritual teacher, and desire to know the highest truth. This can happen because the patient is so to speak in agony.

Kṛṣṇa in the Gītā does, it is true, say (IV.1–3), 'I have taught you this Yoga', but he makes it clear that it is not the human personality that is the teacher. For verse 1 has said: 'I taught this at the beginning of Creation', a declaration of the Cosmic Self as the teacher. As yet, Arjuna finds this impossible to believe.

The next point is that the Gītā here, as in other places, makes a distinction between merely knowing texts and ideas, and seeing the truth in oneself. In the Gītā, Knowledge (jñāna) normally means full realization of the supreme Self. But in a few places, the word for knowledge (jñāna) is paired with a word such as

Realization (vijñāna) or Yoga (identity-meditation, when all senses are inoperative). In those places, Śaṅkara explains that knowledge (jñāna) means intellectual understanding in the form of ideas, as against direct experience beyond ideas. For instance, in VII.1 and 2, the Lord says he will teach, to a yogin, jñāna and its vijñāna. Śaṅkara explains a yogin as one who practises bringing the mind to samādhi-meditation on the Lord; jñāna is knowledge as an idea, whereas vijñāna is being-that-oneself (sva-anubhava). In XVI.1 the attributes of seekers after Brahman are listed, and among them is steadiness in Knowledge and yoga. Śaṅkara says that here Knowledge (jñāna) means grasping what the holy texts and the teacher say about the Self, whereas yoga means to realize it in one's own self by withdrawal of the senses and one-pointed concentration. Steadiness he explains as niṣṭhā or firm establishment.

In IV.34 above, the Gītā is similarly distinguishing text-knowers from those who not only know but also directly see the truth (tattva-darśana). It is only these last, says Śaṅkara, who will be able to teach realization to others.

They teach, and the pupil is to learn. In IV.34, the first verse of the group, he is told to learn by bowing, by being attentive, and by asking questions. But the verse cannot be read in isolation. It is part of the group. As Śaṅkara points out, these three things are only external, and they may be done deceptively. He uses a strong word, māyā-vi-tva, which means something like the trickiness of a magician.

Our teacher told us of an incident at a temple in the Himālayas, where a small image of the god Shiva had long been installed in the dim shrine and worshipped as a symbol of God. A European explorer happened to visit the temple, and he said that he felt a magical attraction to it. In fact he gave up his travels, and remained at the shrine as a worshipper of Shiva. He did some service to the shrine, and became well known and respected for his one-pointed devotion. 'He has fallen in love with our Shiva,' remarked the priest. After some months he told them that he now had to return, but begged to be allowed to take the image of Shiva with him. He made a generous donation to the temple to replace it with any other they chose. The priest, impressed by his devotion, agreed, knowing he could easily get another one. Much later they heard that the Shiva image had been carved from a rare jade. Perhaps one of the early kings had commissioned it from China, and then on his deathbed left it to the temple. The explorer knew about jades, and even in the dim light had recognized what it was. Having secured possession of it by his show of devotion, he sold it for a fortune. It had been indeed a magician's trick of illusion.

The three external means – obeisance, questioning and service – can thus be imitated. There is an Eastern saying: 'Beware of slaves.' This is not in the sense of the Roman maxim: 'As many slaves you have, you have that number of enemies.' The Eastern saying is more profound. The slave does everything for his master, even things which the master can do easily himself. Gradually it is the slave who knows where things are, and what to do when something unexpected turns up. The master finds the slave more and more useful. Finally the slave is not merely useful, but essential. He has taken over the running of everything. The master, though accorded every respect and flattery, is in fact overshadowed by the slave, 'as the god is overshadowed by the priest who outwardly worships him'. The slave has in fact become the master. Some of the Roman emperors were manipulated in this way by their freed men, who had been their slaves.

The climb from slave to master is not necessarily conscious. At first, it may be a naïve self-deception. For a century the royal house of Nepal were kept confined to the palace grounds, surrounded with enervating luxury. The hereditary chief ministers ran the country, keeping the royal family absolutely free from cares, as they put it. There have been similar cases in Chinese history, where the phrase for it is 'prisoners of Heaven'. The rule by the devoted 'slaves' is autocratic and tyrannical: they claim to be slaves themselves, so no one else can be allowed to be anything more than a slave – to them.

Dr Shastri quotes his own teacher as saying: 'serve without being slavish'. Śaṅkara on Gītā II.48 makes the acute comment that the devotee should feel that he is doing the action as an agent of the Lord, but without any idea 'may the Lord be pleased with it'. If this last thought accompanies the action, the mind will be disturbed. Should some outside event make the action fail, the agent will tend to think: 'Well this was done purely as an offering to the Lord. Surely he might have protected it. Is the Lord being ungrateful?' The diaries even of future saints record such thoughts. Śaṅkara says that it is essential to rise above them by practising the yoga of even-mindedness.

These three – reverence, questioning and service – are normally the external means, though in an emergency they can be largely dispensed with. What are the inner and direct means to attain Knowledge, and from Knowledge, freedom? They are briefly given at Chapter IV. 38 and 39:

> There is no purifier in the world like knowledge; the one who is perfected in Yoga will in time himself find it in himself. ....

> The man of faith gets knowledge, intent on it, restraining the senses; having attained knowledge, in no long time he goes to peace.

As often in the Gītā, the instruction (in verse 38) seems to go in a circle. It begins by praising Knowledge as the supreme purifier, then goes on to say that, to get Knowledge, you have to be perfected in yoga. But perfection in yoga itself depends on purification, as the Gītā points out again and again. In this and other cases, the idea is that the process will be gradual at first, because the taints to be removed show themselves as real. Through the methods of yoga, the major taints of attachment, anger, inertia and so on are removed piecemeal, for instance by meditating on the opposite of each in turn. The rise of Knowledge however shows them up as illusions, and so can sweep away any remainder in one stroke. Śaṅkara elsewhere compares it to laundering. They first remove the major patches of grime from the cloths separately, but finally immerse the cloths wholesale in the cleansing vat.

The process of yoga in verse 38 is explained by Śaṅkara as karma-yoga and samādhi-yoga. He is repeating his analysis of karma-yoga under II.39. Samādhi-yoga is the most refined part of karma-yoga; he says that the perfection consists of purification, and becoming able to desire release.

Such a true seeker will 'in time' – after long practice of the yoga, says Śaṅkara – 'himself find it in himself'. This sentence, as many others, shows that though the teacher teaches about the Self, it has to be found by the pupil himself, in himself. He cannot get it from another. It is the Lord who wakens in his own self, as the Self, annihilating all distinctions of individual self and others. For this reason the Gītā does not recommend a pupil to practise helplessness in the form 'What can I do, worthless as I am?' Though it may be provisionally true of the individual body-mind-ego complex, man himself is not that complex. Conviction of helplessness, as the Muṇḍaka Upaniṣad says, is turning away from the splendour of the Lord within. 'It cannot be attained by the one without strength.'

The truth-seeing teacher teaches, but the learner realizes it in himself by himself. This phrase 'in himself by himself' comes often in the Gītā. 'By meditation, some see the Self in the self by the self' (XIII.24).

Verse 39 of Chapter IV here gives a summary of the qualification, process and goal. It is one of the places where Śaṅkara of his own accord states the essentials for finding Knowledge. He is singling it out as a central teaching in the light of which others are to be read.

> The man of faith gets Knowledge. Intent on it, restraining the senses: having attained Knowledge, in no long time he goes to peace.

Faith is applied to the other means: faith in the holy texts, faith in the teacher's presentation of them, faith in the methods of yoga, and faith in the goal. Faith has not only the ordinary meaning of firm belief, but a special meaning of steady commitment to a decision once taken. It is assumed that the decision has been taken after considering the different factors. Even so, nearly everyone experiences a weakening of resolve after doing some practice. It takes the form: 'Well, after all, how do we know? It may be a waste of time, it may be unsettling, it may be dangerous, it may be a swindle.' No new facts have appeared; it is just a sort of re-shuffling of ideas. At that time the spiritual will, technically called faith, says: 'No! We have been into all that, and we made our decision. Now we will keep to it.'

The man of faith will persist and finally attain. But (Śaṅkara comments) he may be very slow. While things are comfortable, he may think: 'I will do it, but later on'. So there is another requirement: 'intent on it' (tat-parah). It is literally, 'putting that above all', so it means that the drive for Knowledge must be the first priority. Dr Shastri's teacher, Shri Dada, like the Buddha, left his home when family pressure made it impossible to pursue the quest there. But this is not a rule: Shri Dada returned to a home life after his training, whereas the Buddha never again set up a home. In the Gītā, Arjuna, a married man, is not recommended to leave family life. But 'tat-parah' does mean to be independent of anything in the world, and to be able to demonstrate that independence if necessary

Intensity of search must invigorate all the other elements of yoga, external or internal. Dr Shastri said: Do not run to serve and serve blindly: seek to know the true nature of man and the universe. Again, without intensity of search, meditation can easily drift into mere dreaming, where there is no change and none is expected.

The last of the three essentials is restraining the senses. The classical example is given in II.58. As a tortoise withdraws its limbs into its shell, so the meditator must withdraw the senses. (The same simile is given by St Teresa of Avila, with the comment: 'Whoever it was that said this, doubtless knew what he was talking about.') There are countless references to the process in the Gītā, often by the word 'yukta'. This comes from the same root as 'yoga'; and could be translated yoked-in-meditation. In many cases Śaṅkara explains it as samādhi or samāhita-citta.

This is not the same meditation practice as in some Buddhist sects, in which awareness of surroundings is retained, but inner reactions to them are minimal. In the yogic meditation the senses ultimately do not function at all. They are, so to speak, asleep. If the meditation is light, they can be roused by a strong stimulus. But in the deep samādhi, the withdrawal is not disturbed by anything external. On this point it is similar to what is called trance and Dr Shastri occasionally so translated it for such cases.

The working of the triple process – faith, intensity and meditation are illustrated briefly in Śaṅkara's two commentaries to the Kena Upaniṣad. An advanced pupil, confident in his knowledge of truth, is told by his teacher: 'If you think you know it, little indeed you know'. The pupil, shaken, goes to sit in a solitary place, and concentrates in samādhi on the text 'I am Brahman'. He has to bring to a unity the ideas learned from the texts and teacher, with the different ideas of what he actually experiences. He has till now tacitly accepted the difference, making it disappear like a sort of vanishing conjuring trick. But now he has to press the point, calling on all his resources of courage. Finally the needle-point of concentration pierces through the 'I' of the text to the reality beyond it. He comes back to the teacher, saying: 'I do not think "I know", but it is not that I do not know.' The Upaniṣad confirms this with the verse: 'Unknown to those who know; known to those who do not know.'

In the same way, Zen teachers sometimes give riddles. Here an impossibility is often clear from the outset. 'What was your original face before your mother was born?' The Koan riddle is solved only on a trans-personal basis. To think or say 'I have solved it' is a personal assertion which shows that the koan has not been passed through. Nor does a teacher ever say: 'You have solved it.'

In many mystical traditions, a current appears from time to time to the effect that the statement of truth must be sufficient. All subsidiary methods such as meditation are less-than-truth, and so untruth, and so obstacles. Such schools die out in a few generations, as did the Zen school of Shen-hui in China which turned into theoretical philosophy. As to why they give up meditation practice, there are various reasons. One of them may be in a remark by a young British abstract painter. Asked why he had rejected representational art with its rules of perspective and so on, he answered briefly: 'Couldn't do it.'

Bukko, the great Chinese Zen master who inspired the Japanese rulers to repulse the Mongol invasions at the end of the thirteenth century, was asked by a scholar: 'We have the truth handed down by Buddhas and patriarchs. How should any "way" be required?' Bukko replied: 'The seeds have indeed been sown, but the shoots do not appear.' He explained no further. Zen teachers do not like to explain. The saying is, 'If I hold up one corner and he cannot come back with the other three, I do not teach him further.' We are left to infer that if the ground has not been broken up and the stones and weeds removed, the seeds will not germinate. The ground, so to say, cannot take them.

It can be the same on the mental planes. In 1982, Aspect in Paris made the first experimental verification of non-locality, and necessary involvement of consciousness, on the quantum level in physics. It was a conclusion against which Einstein and Schrödinger had fought: they hated the implications of the quantum physics they had helped to found. Einstein said bluntly: 'I refuse to believe that an ant changes the universe by looking at it.'

Again, he made his famous remark: 'God does not play dice with the universe.' To which the answer came: 'How does he know?'

As has been pointed out, there should have been an earthquake in science, but in fact there was not. To provide a conceptual basis for the results 'stretches the human imagination further than it can go; the pointer is neither up nor down, but somehow hovers in between'. In fact no scientist believes it except a few physicists. And this is not so unreasonable, because there do not seem to be any immediate consequences. Things still work. As Ernst Mach in Prague held over a century ago, the job of science is not to tell us truth, but to show us how to make things work, so that we can use them for our lives.

Somehow – apparently under the control of consciousness – the uncertainties of the quantum level become certainties of ordinary experience, which are assumed to be 'out there, independent of consciousness'. There is a tacit agreement to ignore the recent developments. Lip-service may be paid, but the mind simply cannot take them in.

In the same way in Vedānta, the texts may be known, but not taken in. As an instance of it, look at the Gītā itself. A main teaching in its eighteen chapters is that the world is the māyā of the Lord. The Gītā declares itself as given on a battlefield, awaiting the signal to begin. It ends when the signal is given.

One may imagine the following conversation:

> 'It takes me at least two hours to read aloud the Gītā. The two armies couldn't have waited that long: historically, it just couldn't happen'.
>
> 'Could it happen in a dream?'
>
> 'Oh, in a dream yes. It could happen in a dream'.

'This is the dream'.

The Gītā at the end of Chapter II declares that this waking world is night for the sage who sees. Śaṅkara explains this as like a dream, and (elsewhere) like a mirage, like a castle in the sky and like other illusions. They have practical reality (thirsty travellers make for a mirage), following laws on their own. Nevertheless there is an instinctive rejection of the idea that the whole world-experience is as an illusion; the texts say it, but the mind cannot take them in.

So the three essential methods – faith, intensity of search and withdrawal-meditation – are necessary. The three external methods, such as attendance on a teacher, are natural expressions of faith. They become genuine when they express intensity of search.

If we look through the Gītā, we see that Arjuna does come to get the requirements for yoga. Some of them appear only after the terrible shock of Chapter XI. His faith develops from the incredulity of IV.4 to the reverence and prostration of XI.44. His questions change from the personal 'Which shall I do?' (II.7 – though immediately followed by 'I will not fight') to intense search for truth (X.16) in meditation (X.17). When yoga is matured, the yogin finds Knowledge in himself by himself, or as X.15 puts it, the Lord knows himself by himself.

The teacher in the Gītā is the universal Lord, the supreme Self. As Chapter X declares, that universal Self takes on limited divine forms such as Rāma, Kṛṣṇa, Yama, god of death, Kandarpa, god of love, Skanda, god of death, and also the forms of human teachers such as Vyāsa, compiler of the Vedas. What is the role of the human teacher, the Knower and the Truth-seer of IV.34? He explains the holy texts, and answers questions on them.

But there is something more, best perhaps described symbolically. The saying in the yogic schools is: 'You cannot see the dirt on your own face.' The yogin purifies his body and mind by the methods of yoga under the direction of the teacher. He is aware of the taints, and works hard to remove them. But there remains a small piece of dirt which he does not know about, because it is so close to him. This is the dirt on one's own face. It is the teacher who takes up a clean cloth when the pupil presents himself face-to-face. Then a gentle wipe, wipe – and the true universal face shines forth, as it was before Mother World-illusion was born.

Rebirth

> II.22 As the wearer casts off worn-out clothes and puts on himself others which are new,
> Even so, casting off worn-out bodies, the body-wearer passes on to new ones.

This great verse on reincarnation comes at the beginning of the teachings, and it refers to the great Self which takes on itself the illusion of the succession of bodies.

A master of meditation remarked that the idea of reincarnation contains hints at wider truths than the bare idea of things wearing out and being replaced, which to many older people has a depressing ring. They find their bodies less and less reliable, and less competent to fulfil most of the purposes of life as they have understood them. He said:

> 'Take the case of furniture. If a chair is reasonably well made, at the beginning it sparkles with the fresh varnish laid evenly all over it. It has an unyielding firmness, and is

perfectly adapted for its purpose. But it is not necessarily particularly attractive. Now suppose it has been in use for a hundred years. A good deal of the varnish will have been rubbed off the arms where the sitter has let himself down. For some years it was very comfortable as it gave slightly to the movements of the body, but in the end the whole thing got somewhat rickety. Now it has to be sat on with extreme care, and perhaps finally not at all. If it has been polished and polished for so long, the glare of the new varnish will have become a subdued glow. The chair is from the practical point of view almost useless, but as a matter of fact it is highly appreciated. It diffuses a soft radiance all around; it may even become a valuable antique.

'In the same way a personality, if it has been used properly and polished every day by meditation, may become less active in the affairs of the world, but it spreads an atmosphere of quiet peace. It too has a sort of subdued radiance.

'It is not quite the same with clothes, which don't after all become antiques. But in fact old clothes are generally much more comfortable than new ones; they have come to adapt to the body. When we are wearing new clothes, we generally are not quite at ease. We take care that not a speck of anything drops on them, and we don't care to go out even for a moment into rain. Whereas with the old clothes, though it is true that we handle them with care too, it is done with a kind of affection and without any worry. When they are finally laid aside, we give a little thought of gratitude for their faithful service. And it can be the same with the personality when it is time for that too to be laid aside.

> 'In this way we can bring meaning to the whole of the incarnation in which we find ourself, instead of thinking of it as just the first part, with the later parts as without real meaning.'

Spiritual life can and should grow stronger every year!

Play

Yoga sees another causality underlying the causality of the world. A stage play has its own causal sequence: within the play, daggers kill, kings are honoured, the mother loves a baby. But there is a deeper causal sequence which is quite different: the daggers do not kill though the stabbed man falls, the king is a very minor role, the baby over which the mother croons is a doll. All the events, though they seem determined by the stage situation, are in fact free choices by the cast. They are careful to preserve the play situation. They do not lean against a pillar in the palace; if someone did, a ripple would go across the marble of the painted scenery. A keen eye can in fact see many of the inconsistencies in the stage setting and action of the play, though children are often completely deceived.

In something of the same way, yoga sees the cosmos as controlled and held together by intelligence. Sometimes its particular functions are called deva-s, or shining ones, or gods. They may be directly perceived by some yogins who worship God in his manifestations. Śaṅkara states in one of his commentaries that ancient sages met the gods face to face, and it can be the same today for those who meditate on them through yoga. But the Gītā expects the yogin finally to look deeper than outer divine manifestation, and find the Lord within himself also. The Lord is so to say the producer of the play.

One may feel: 'All the talk about the divine in Nature is very well while things go well, while it is a question of beautiful scenery and good health and so on. But what about when things are really bad? Can even the most advanced yogin retain his vision then?'

As an introduction, here is an account of an incident in the life of Swami Rama Tirtha, once a fellow disciple of Dr Shastri. He was a totally dedicated yogin, even during his worldly career as a Professor of Mathematics, and this state showed itself while he was still a young man. It would take one of milder resolution and training efforts a much longer time. But the mahatma said that it would be reached by all who persisted.

The Procession

A great mahātma, Rama Tirtha, after his God-realization found he could no longer continue a home life in society, as Professor of Mathematics at Lahore University. He went to live at great heights in the Himalayas, occasionally coming down to give talks and publish articles. On one such occasion his former teacher sent a young brahmacari to look after him.

One day the mahātma gave a four-hour long discourse to an audience of thousands; he danced on the sands of the Ganges, and many of the audience saw a god there dancing.

Afterwards he went back with the brahmacari to the small room where he was staying. The mahātma's lack of interest in food and his solitary life in the mountains had upset his digestive system, and he sometimes suffered from attacks of colic. When the spasms came on, his body twisted and turned. The disciple watched with horror, and when he found there was nothing he could do to help he burst into tears.

The mahātma patted him on the head and said: 'My son, Rama is above all this.'

'But when you danced, we saw a god dancing there,' sobbed the brahmacari, 'and .... How can this happen to you?'

The mahātma replied; 'You know the procession of Rama when it goes through the village, don't you? What a joyous occasion it is! The image of the god passes, so majestic, so exalting; then the band and its music, and some of the devotees singing the songs of divine love. Then come the acrobats, some distance behind the palanquin of the god, displaying their skill to take part in this great occasion. And finally there are the clowns, aren't there? They turn somersaults to amuse the children and to add to the general happiness. You know all this, and you appreciate it all.

'The same thing is happening here: it is a divine procession through the body of Rama. The dance on the sands – that was the passing of the god before your eyes. And now, following the procession, here are the acrobats and the clowns, making their bodies twist and turn. It is all the divine procession, and Rama is an onlooker, appreciating it.'

Part V

Technical Appendices

Introductory

Except where otherwise stated, the reference to a Gītā verse is in fact to Śaṅkara's commentary on that verse.

There are many cases where Śaṅkara comments on a verse from a distance; in other words, in his commentary to another verse, not necessarily nearby, or previous. For instance, an important anticipatory comment to VII.16–18 appears already under IV.11.

The present appendix is not a study, but a collection of a few texts to illustrate some central points of Gītā practice as Śaṅkara sees it.

1 Translation of Śaṅkara's Introduction to the Gītā

Nārāyaṇa is beyond the Unmanifest;
From the Unmanifest the cosmic Egg comes to be.
And within the Egg are the cosmic regions,
And the earth of seven continents.

Having thus projected the world (jagat), to stabilize it the Lord first projected Marīci and others as lords of creation, and directed them to what the Veda calls the Right Course (dharma) of Engagement-in-action.

Then he brought forth others like Sanaka and Sanandana, and directed them to the Right Course of Cessation-from-action, consisting of Knowledge (jñāna) and Detachment (vairāgya).

Thus the Vedic Course is two-fold: Engagement-in-action, and Cessation-from-action.

The stability of the world is based on this two-fold Course, which directly produces for its beings relative prosperity and Absolute Good respectively. It is practised by those of the Brahmin and other classes, in their various stages of life, who seek their good.

But over a long time, with the rise of desire in the practisers, the Right Course became overcome by the Wrong Course which flourished by reducing their discrimination and knowledge. Then to restore the world order, the First Creator Viṣṇu, here called Nārāyaṇa, to preserve the immanence of Brahman-on-earth, cast a ray of himself through Vasudeva into Devakī, and came to be the child Kṛṣṇa.

For by preservation of the Brahmin spirit of truth, the whole divine Course would be preserved, from which the classes and stages of life are derived.

So the Lord, of eternal omniscience, supremacy, potentiality (śakti), power, energy, and glory directed his own divine (vaiṣṇava) trick-of-illusion (māyā), of three guṇa-elements, which is called root-Nature (mūla-prakṛti). And though himself unborn, unchanging, and ever pure, aware, and free, by his own māyā-illusion He is taken to be a body-wearer as it were, born as it were, giving to the world his grace as it were.

With no purpose of his own to serve but solely for the sake of living beings, he taught the holy two-fold Course to Arjuna, then sunk in a sea of grief and delusion. For a Course will spread when accepted and practised by those of outstanding character.

The Course thus taught by the Lord was set out by the omniscient sage Vyāsa, compiler of the Veda-s, in seven hundred verses, famous as the Gītā. It is however difficult to realize how this Gītā scripture is the whole essence of the Veda teaching.

Though there have been some who have tried to make it clear by analysing the make-up and sense of the individual words and sentences, I have found that it has been taken in absolutely opposite ways by people at large. So I propose to make a brief commentary (vivaraṇa) to determine the meaning accurately.

Briefly, the purport of this Gītā scripture is, the Supreme Good (niḥśreyasa), and the means to it – namely absolute cessation of the world-flow (saṃsāra) and its cause. This comes about through following the Course of Establishment-in-Knowledge (jñāna-niṣṭhā) as following on the casting off (saṃnyāsa) of all action (karma).

This very Course, the purport of the Gītā, has been taught by the Lord in the words of the Anu-Gītā verses:

> 'This Course (dharma) easily suffices for realization of Brahman' (Mahābh.Aśva.16.12)

and again

> 'neither righteous nor sinful, neither good nor bad' (*ibid.* 19.7)

> 'who sits alone and silent, in one posture, thinking nothing' (*ibid.* 19.1)

> 'knowledge with saṃnyāsa' (*ibid.* 4.3.25).

In the present Gītā too Arjuna is told:

> 'Having given up all action, resort to Me alone' (XVIII.66).

Though the Course which looks for relative good, namely Engagement-in-Action with its classes and stages of life, has also been taught as a means to attain such things as heavenly realms, still when performed as an offering to the Lord, it comes to be for purification-of-essence (sattva-śuddhi), no longer bound to results. A pure essence also acts as a means to the Highest Good by way of attaining the capacity for Establishment-in-Knowledge (jñāna-niṣṭhā), and by causing the first rise of that Knowledge. And so it will be said: 'Consigning all actions to Brahman' (V.10) and 'The yogins do actions without attachment to purify themselves' (V.11).

The Gītā scripture has for its subject: the two-fold Course with the Highest Good (niḥśreyasa) as its purpose, and the transcendental truth known as Vāsudeva. It explains them in detail in terms of definite subject-matter, a purpose, and the connection between them. To realize it is to fulfil the whole purpose of man, and this is why I now undertake the task of composing a commentary (vivaraṇa) on it.

2 Jñāna-Yoga Path for Sāṅkhya-s (=Knowers) from Śaṅkara Gītā Commentary

II.21 The Knower (jñānin) has nothing to do with action.
(Question) What then has he to do?
(Answer) This is answered in III.3: 'The Sāṅkhya-s should resort to jñāna-yoga.'

For the Knower and seeker of Liberation, who sees that the Self is actionless, there is qualification for renunciation-of-all-action alone (avikriyātma-darśino viduṣo mumukṣo ca sarva-karma-saṃnyāse eva adhikāra).

II.55 The Knower (vidvat), having renounced, makes efforts in jñāna-niṣṭhā.

The above quotations illustrate the path of Knowledge-yoga (jñāna-yoga). It begins with the rise of Knowledge, which distinguishes the Sāṅkhya. The path consists of (1) renunciation-of-action (saṃnyāsa): this renunciation is not necessarily of things, but is characterized as freedom from the notion 'I do'; (2) establishment-in-Knowledge (jñāna-niṣṭhā), sustained meditations to throw off disturbances, by memory-illusions, of the naturally continuing current of Knowledge. When jñāna-niṣṭhā reaches its end (avasāna) in being-Brahman (anubhava), it is Freedom (mokṣa).

Here follow a few passages to illustrate Śaṅkara's scheme. He does not spell out all the stages each time: for instance, saṃnyāsa may include jñāna-niṣṭhā.

	Rise of Knowledge	Saṃnyāsa	Jñāna-niṣṭhā	Mokṣa
II.10,11	self-knowledge (ātma-jña) jñānin=Sāṅkhya	saṃnyāsa jñāna-yoga		end of saṃsāra
21	seer of Self (ātma-darśin)	saṃnyāsa		
21	Knower=vidvat = Sāṅkhya	saṃnyāsa by mind (5.13)		
54,55	vidvat samādhi-stha	saṃnyāsa	jñāna-yoga-niṣṭhā (2.56–72)	Brahman
69	ātma-jña	saṃnyāsa	jñāna-niṣṭhā	
III intro.	jñāna	saṃnyāsa	jñāna-niṣṭhā	
III.3	Sāṅkhya =ātma-jña	saṃnyāsa	jñāna-niṣṭhā	Goal
III.4	rise of Knowledge		jñāna-niṣṭhā	
17	Sāṅkhya Self-knower	saṃnyāsin	ātma-jñāna-niṣṭhā	
IV.39	jñāna-labha		quickly	mokṣa
V intro.	ātma-tattva-vid		jñāna-yoga-niṣṭhā	
	Self-knower	saṃnyāsa		
	Sāṅkhya	saṃnyāsin	jñāna-niṣṭhā	
	jñāna	saṃnyāsa		siddhi (perfection)
V.4	Sāṅkhya-Knower	saṃnyāsa		
5	Sāṅkhya	saṃnyāsin	jñāna-niṣṭhā	mokṣa
6	paramātma-jñāna	paramārthaka-saṃnyāsa	paramātma-jñāna-niṣṭhā	
12	jñāna-prāpti	sarva-karma-saṃnyāsa	jñāna-niṣṭhā	peace mokṣa
13	paramārtha-darśin; vidvat	mental saṃnyāsa	rests happy	
17	Sāṅkhya (Ś.2.69)		jñāna-niṣṭhā	live in Brahman
25	samyag-darśin	saṃnyāsa		Brahma-nirvāṇa
26,27	samyag-darśana jñāna-prāpti	saṃnyāsa	samyag-darśana-niṣṭhā	mokṣa
VII.16–18	jñānin tattva-vid		samādhi on I am Vāsudeva	comes to Me
19	jñāna-vat		paripāka-jñāna	comes to Me

IX.22	paramārtha-darśin	saṃnyāsin	'Lord as Self' (=jñāna-niṣṭhā, Ś on 18.66)	
X.8	paramārtha-tattva-vid		intense meditation (bhāvana)	
X.10	samyag-darśana		buddhi-yoga	
11	jñāna	withdrawal	dhyāna vision	bliss
XII.4	jñānin	saṃnyāsin	meditation	one with Me
5	paramārtha-darśana		jñāna-niṣṭhā	mokṣa
10	jñāna-prāpti			siddhi
12	samyag-darśin	saṃnyāsa		
13,14	jñānin (of 7.17) mumukṣu (12.19)	saṃnyāsa	jñāna-niṣṭhā	immortality
XIII.31	paramārtha-darśin=Sāṅkhya	paramahaṃsa parivrājaka	jñāna-niṣṭhā	
XIV.1	jñāna	saṃnyāsa	manana-śīla	mokṣa
23–25	ātma-vid = Sāṅkhya (3.5)	saṃnyāsin	mumukṣu	
26,27		saṃnyāsin	jñāna-niṣṭhā jñāna-yoga	mokṣa
XVIII.3	tattva-vid = Sāṅkhya	perceives no pain in Self	meditate: 'I do nothing'	
10	jñāna	mind-saṃnyāsa	jñāna-niṣṭhā	
12	paramārtha-darśin	paramahaṃsa parivrājaka	kevala-samyag-darśana-niṣṭhā	end of saṃsāra
45,46			jñāna-niṣṭhā	
49	jñāna	mind-saṃnyāsa	jñāna-niṣṭhā = naiṣkarmyasiddhi	mokṣa

3 Niṣṭhā

Śaṅkara's doctrine of liberation in the Gītā is set out briefly in his introduction: the Highest good ... is from the Course (dharma) of Establishment-in-Knowledge-of-Self (ātma-jñāna-niṣṭhā), preceded by completely casting off all action (sarva-karma-saṃnyāsa). He presents it at length at the end, in the commentary to XVIII.50, 54, and 55, in the following extracts:

XVIII.50

That supreme establishment-in-Knowledge (niṣṭhā jñānasya yā parā niṣṭhā) is its final resting-place (pary-avasāna), its culmination (pari-samāpti)

That is the supreme culmination of Knowledge of Brahman (brahma-jñānasya yā parā parisamāpti).

XVIII.54 (extract)

> Such a man of jñāna-niṣṭhā (establishment-in-Knowledge), My devotee (bhakta) worshipping Me the supreme Lord, has attained the fourth, the highest, devotion (bhakti), that which has Knowledge. As it was said
>
> (VII.18) *The fourth class* (the class of Knowers) *worship Me.* So by that bhakti of Knowledge –

XVIII.55 (extract)

> By devotion he knows Me, how great and who I am in truth:
> Then having known Me in truth, he thereupon enters.
>
> (Śaṅkara) *Then having known Me in truth, he thereupon enters* into Me. It is not meant by this that there are two

separate actions – an entering apart from Knowledge. *Having known, he thereupon enters* means Knowledge alone with no further result. So it was said: *Know me as the Knower of the field* (XIII.2).

(Opponent) It is a contradiction to what was said previously (XVIII.50) that what is highest is Establishment (niṣṭhā) of Knowledge, and by that he knows Me. To explain the contradiction: when the Knowledge of something simply arises in a Knower, then the Knower is said to know that thing. He does not look to some establishment, some going over again, of the knowledge. So the contradiction is, that it was said previously that it is not by knowledge but by Establishment-of-Knowledge (jñāna-niṣṭhā), by going over it again that one knows.

(Answer) There is no contradiction, for the force of the word Establishment (niṣṭhā) is, the definite coming-to-rest (avasānatva) in Self-being (ātma-anubhava) of a Knowledge that has met the conditions for its own rise (utpatti) and maturing (paripāka), (namely) absence of obstacles. That is its Establishment (niṣṭhā).

The concomitant conditions for the rise (utpatti) and maturing (paripāka) of the Knowledge from scripture and instruction of a teacher are: purity of buddhi and so on, the (twenty) qualities beginning with humility (XIII.7–11). When from them arises the Knowledge that the Field-Knower (kṣetra-jña) and the highest Self (paramātman) are one, and there is also renunciation of all actions tied up with notions of differences of agent, instruments and so on – when there is thus definite being-the-Self

> (svātma-anubhava) – that state is what is meant by the highest Establishment-of-Knowledge (jñāna-niṣṭhā).
>
> As against the other three types of devotion (bhakti) given in VII.16, namely of those in danger, those seeking Knowledge, or those seeking success in the world, this jñāna-niṣṭhā is called the fourth kind of devotion, the highest. By that highest devotion he knows the Lord in truth. Thereupon, the idea (buddhi) of any difference between the Lord and the Knower of the field, completely ceases. So what is being said is: 'he knows Me in truth by the devotion (bhakti) which is Establishment-in-Knowledge (jñāna-niṣṭhā), and there is no contradiction.

(There follow citations of texts showing that giving up all sense of 'I do' must come before and along with jñāna-niṣṭhā.)

> jñāna-niṣṭhā is unremitting persistence (abhiniveṣa) in the idea-stream of the Self Apart. Bhakti-yoga of serving the Lord by one's proper action has for its perfection this result: becoming capable of jñāna-niṣṭhā. Thus the yoga of bhakti brings about jñāna-niṣṭhā, which has mokṣa as its final resting-place (avasāna). The Lord goes on to praise that yoga in verse 56.

In this short summarizing passage, XVIII.55, Śaṅkara twice distinguishes between the rise (utpatti) of Knowledge and its mature (paripāka) state. Elsewhere he similarly distinguishes Right Vision when it has just arisen (utpanna-samyag-darśana) from its established state (samyag-darśana-niṣṭhā).

The notion of maturing (paripāka) involves time, though not a fixed time. Another key word in the passage is avasāna, which has the sense of a final goal or stage. There is an association with unharnessing horses, or a river finding its bourn in the ocean. He twice refers to the final goal (avasāna) of Knowledge as anubhava. (A separate note on these terms follows.)

As he says in his commentary to V.12, the final stages are (1) sattva-śuddhi (purity of essence), (2) jñāna-prāpti (obtaining Knowledge), (3) saṃnyāsa giving up 'I do' (V.8, and V.13 which is often cited by Śaṅkara in the Gītā commentary on giving up action), (4) jñāna-niṣṭhā, and (5) mokṣa. He calls the whole process krama, meaning a step-by-step progress.

The process of jñāna-niṣṭhā is in fact jñāna-yoga, beginning with Knowledge: it is outlined briefly in XVIII 50–55. Exceptions to the rule of physical renunciation are allowed to kṣatriya Knowers (kṣaṭriyāḥ vidvāṃsāḥ) and others. They are listed in the section called Exceptions.

Jñāna-niṣṭhā is described in the Gītā itself in several places. Śaṅkara gives as main ones:

II.55–72
V.17–26
XII.13–20
XIV.22–25
XVIII.51–54

It is also described shortly in many places. It is concerned not with reinforcing Knowledge, which needs no reinforcement, but with removing obstructions. Such normally arise from prārabdha karma. The instruction to jñāna-niṣṭhā would correspond to an instruction to keep a flowing stream clear, as distinct from creating, or reinforcing, the stream. It is removing any branches that might fall into it, but not pushing the water along, or pouring more in. Normally, some disturbances from prārabdha are to be expected, but there might be none. In some places Śaṅkara gives the brief statement: 'jñāna is the means to mokṣa.' For instance there should be no prārabdha left at the hour of death: it will have come to an end. Knowledge attained at that time has its fruit instantly: it will have no need to 'mature'. So the final hour (as the Gītā and Śaṅkara mention) is specifically favourable.

4 Three Terms

Paripāka (Maturing, Ripening)

Paripāka, having the sense of completion by maturing or ripening, is a feature of Śaṅkara's Gītā presentation. The meaning is that similar, intense saṃskāra-s repeatedly laid down, finally come to dominate the causal or unmanifest basis of the mind. The word 'maturing' implies some passage of time, though it may be very short.

For instance, he says that the Sānkhya-buddhi or knowledge-mind comes about when the karma-yoga-buddhi or action-yoga-mind attains maturity:

> II.49 Have recourse to the karma-yoga buddhi, or to the Sānkhya buddhi which is born when that is mature (tat-paripāka-jāyām).

The Sānkhya-buddhi is only the rise of Knowledge. The Knowledge itself has to mature:

> VII.19 The Knower who has attained mature Knowledge (prāpta-paripāka-jñānam).

Both detachment and meditation have also a process of maturing:

> XVIII.37 The happiness born of the maturing of Knowledge, detachment, meditation and samādhi... is of sattva (jñāna-vairāgya-dhyāna-samādhi-paripāka-jam sukham ... sāttvikam).

Another account of the rise of Knowledge is given in XIII. 11, in the commentary to the twentieth and final quality of those leading to Knowledge, namely tattva-jñāna-artha-darśanam, or Seeing-the-goal-of-Knowledge-of-truth, which goal is mokṣa.

> XIII.11 Knowledge of truth (tattva-jñāna) results from maturity of creative meditation (bhāvanā-paripāka-nimitta) on Humility (amānitva) and the others (ādi) of the group up to the penultimate one, Constancy in Self-Knowledge (adhyātma-jñāna-nityatvam).

Elsewhere the process is referred to by different terms. In the comment on 'strength of yoga' (yoga-bala) under VIII.10, Śaṅkara says:

> the strength of yoga is the fixity of mind arising from accumulation of samskāra-s produced by samādhi (samādhi-ja-saṁskāra-pracaya-janita-citta-sthairya-lakṣaṇa).

(It is noteworthy that Bhāskara, perhaps a near contemporary, who in places of his own Gītā commentary reproduces Śaṅkara, gives this same phrase but without the word samādhi. It is an example of how he avoided the terms of Yoga which Śaṅkara used so plentifully.)

Avasāna (Destination, Resting-Place)

Śaṅkara often uses it to mean the truth into which the illusory appearance is finally resolved.

VIII.3 is a reply to questions by Arjuna, one of which is 'what is adhyātma?' The term has been used in III.30, where Arjuna is told to perform actions 'with mind on the self' (adhyātma-cetasā). At that time he does not know of the Self-as-Brahman, and Śaṅkara there interprets it as the individual self, to be thought of as a servant. Here the Lord explains the term adhyātma as svabhāva, individual selfhood, to be further mentioned in XVII.2. But Śaṅkara adds:

> That self which, overseeing a body, sets out as its inner self, and truly comes to rest (avasāna) as the highest Brahman, is the svabhāva selfhood which is to be called adhy-ātman Selfhood. (Ātmānam deham adhirkṛtya pratyag-ātmatayā pravṛttam paramārtha-Brahmāvasānam vastu svabhāva adhyātmam ucyate).

In IX.10 he says:

> 'I am in pain', 'I will do this', 'I will know that' – is all based on knowledge (avagati-niṣṭhā), (and) comes down to knowledge (avagaty-avasāna).

Anubhava

In the Gītā commentary this means roughly being (bhava) in-accordance-with (anu) what truly is. The sense comes out clearly in III.41 and IX.1, where the Gītā has the pair jñāna-vijñāna. (This is translated by Edgerton as theoretical and practical knowledge.) In this pairing, jñāna is taken by Śaṅkara not in the usual way as Right Vision (samyag-darśana), but as theoretical ideas (ava-bodha) of the Self and so on as taught by scripture and the teacher. Vijñāna in contrast is practical realization of the ideas – anubhava.

Similarly in IX.1 vijñāna as anubhava is distinguished from jñāna. But he also treats the pair together as samyagdarśana, 'the direct means to mokṣa'.

The Three Terms: Paripāka, Avasāna, Anubhava

The three terms – paripāka, avasāna, anubhava – came together (each twice) in XVIII.55. They also appear under XVIII.36 and 37.

The Gītā and Śaṅkara both treat the teaching-point here as most important: Kṛṣṇa introduces it with Hear!, which Śaṅkara glosses as: Be Concentrated (samādhānam kuru).

> XVIII.36 Hear from me about the three-fold happiness.

> What with practice one delights in, where pain comes to an end,
> XVIII.37 Which at the beginning seems like poison but with maturity is like honey.
> That is said to be the happiness of light (sattva),
> Arising from the peace of a mind-resting-on-Self (ātmabuddhi).

'with practice' means by application and facility; 'delight' means happiness-realization (sukha-anubhava). He does not use anubhava for the momentary experience of false happiness of excitement or the deluded happiness of sloth.

Śaṅkara explains that at the beginning, when jñāna, vairāgya, dhyāna and samādhi are first tackled head-on, they are nothing but effort; in this preliminary stage, they seem against natural well-being – poison as it were. But when the jñāna, vairāgya, dhyāna and samādhi are mature (paripāka) the happiness is comparable to honey of immortality.

5 Karma-Yoga

The terms yoga and karma-yoga are occasionally used interchangeably by Śaṅkara, especially contrasted with the jñāna-yoga of Sāṅkhya. He defines Yoga in II.39.

Yoga, the means to that (Knowledge), is (1) first, distancing oneself (reading prahāna with Ānandagiri and not prahanana 'killing') from the pairs- of-opposites (dvandva); (2) undertaking actions as karma-yoga, namely as worship (ārādhana) of God; (3) samādhi-yoga.

In IV.38, 'purified by yoga' is glossed as purified by karma-yoga and samādhi-yoga. The accompanying word mumukṣu presumably would cover dvandva-prahāna.

In XII.12 and elsewhere, karma-yoga is used as yoga, to include other elements besides action:

> Yoga is said to be samādhi – concentration on the Lord (īśvare cetah-samādhāna), and a performance for the Lord's sake of actions, and so on. It rests on seeing difference between Self (ātman) and the Lord (ātmeṣvara bheda āsritya) It is not compatible with Right Vision (samyag-darśana-ananvita).... It relies on an Īśvara apart. So Jñāna-yoga, which knows the Lord to be the Self, is not practicable for a karma-yogin.... Conversely, the jñāna-yogin, who sees no difference between them, would have no incentive to rely on a supposedly purely external Lord.

Nevertheless, though (as Śaṅkara points out) the Lord directs Arjuna (in IV. 15) to karma-yoga, this is after his first teaching of Jñāna, in Chapter II, has had no effect. Jñāna yoga has been taught to Arjuna, but he could not then follow it.

In X.19 the Lord specifically consents to Arjuna's request, by declaring: 'I will tell you of my glories.' For constant meditation (nitya dhyeya) says Śaṅkara, and adds: 'Listen!' The first of these glories is: 'I am the Self (aham ātmā) in every living being,' which is a statement of jñāna. Then, for one who cannot meditate on the Lord as Self (tad-asakta), the glories of the Lord immanent in Māyā are given.

Later in X.37 it is even more direct: 'I am Dhanañjaya' (Arjuna), but Arjuna fails to take it in (though for a moment he thinks he has). So in fact instruction in jñāna is given, but while Arjuna's basic feeling is that of karma-yoga, he cannot be rightly said to be on the jñāna-yoga path.

6 Saṃnyāsa

To enter the order of saṃnyāsa was to leave home and property and wander forth, sustained by semi-automatic actions of body-mind like begging and lying down to sleep and so on. Śaṅkara cites three times in his Gītā commentary the Bṛhad. Up. III.5.1: 'Having known (viditvā) that Self, they wander forth as mendicants.'

Śaṅkara, like the Gītā itself, is against physical renunciations while there is inner longing for objects: in his lead-in to Gītā III.6 he says: 'For one who does not know the Self, it is not-right (asat) that he should not undertake his required duty.'

For the Self-knower (Sāṅkhya, jnānin, tattva-vid, samyag-darśin, etc.) on the other hand, voluntarily initiated actions will tend to drop away, with the desires that cause them. Saṃnyāsa will tend to follow naturally upon Knowledge. Nevertheless Śaṅkara very frequently enjoins it as a necessary accessory to Knowledge: it then leads to Establishment-in-Knowledge (jñāna-niṣṭhā) and finally Liberation (mokṣa). In the Gītā commentary he makes the essence of saṃnyāsa to be: giving up the notion (pratyaya) of 'I do.'

In places he describes saṃnyāsa as being in fact jñāna-niṣṭhā. For instance, under XVIII.12 he calls the highest saṃnyāsin, the paramahaṃsa parivrājaka, kevala-jñāna-niṣṭhā and kevala-samyag-darśana-niṣṭha. He often uses the term saṃnyāsa to include both. The samṇyāsa order was usually spoken of in relation to Brahmins, but in XVIII.45 and 46 he states that all classes can qualify themselves for jñāna-niṣṭhā by carrying out their proper duty with devotion.

In the Gītā commentary, Śaṅkara refers to five kinds of saṃnyāsa:

1. *saṃnyāsa as outer show*. In this the property and home are renounced, but no attempt is made at inner renunciation. In India, sometimes a well-off man expecting to die would, just before the end, give away everything in order to get merit in the future. (But sometimes he embarrassingly recovered.) See also the opening of the Kaṭha Upaniṣad. Others took to the anonymous wandering life to escape family, creditors, or police. All this is condemned by the Gītā (e.g. III.6).
2. *Partial saṃnyāsa*, where only some actions and things are renounced. This renouncer still feels 'I do', and is still affected by the results of his actions. He simply reduces them. Śaṅkara refers to this without approval (intro, to V), and remarks that it is 'difficult', as needing great self-control.
3. *Honorary saṃnyāsa*, where things and actions are not given up, but only attachment to them and their fruits. The agent still feels 'I do.' This is a main element of karma yoga.
4. *saṃnyāsa by Mind*, which is renunciation by a Truth-knower (tattva-vid, samyag-darśin, etc.). The Gītā directs him to constant meditation with concentrated mind (samāhita citta) on 'I do nothing', though undertakings continue to be carried out by the body and

mind. Onlookers suppose they are performed by an individual as before.

5. *Supreme (paramārtha) renunciation.* Its essential quality is the meditation 'I do nothing', but this is now reflected outwardly in physical withdrawal into the order of paramahaṃsa-parivrājaka, wandering mendicants.

7 Exceptions to Formal Saṃyāsa

In Gītā III.20 and IV.15 it is said that Janaka and other ancient worthies sought perfection through action alone. Śaṅkara, with his emphasis on Liberation (perfection) through Knowledge alone, has to meet objections based on these texts. Commenting on Gītā II.11, where the teachings begin, he says:

> Those of them who were Knowers of truth (tattva-vid) had sought their perfection by Knowledge alone and had now reached the stage of formal saṃnyāsa: but as Kṣatriya kings they would have been already involved in actions. So realizing 'it is guṇa-s acting on guṇa-s', they continued in action for the sake of the other people (loka-saṅgraha), to fulfil their past karmic involvement (prārabdhatvāt), though they were seeking perfection of Liberation through their Knowledge alone.
>
> Those of them who were not yet Knowers sought perfection through action for self-purification and (then) rise of Knowledge.

Śaṅkara explains away the phrase 'by action alone' in III.20 by glossing it as 'not giving up action'. He also cites the 'thus knowing' of IV.15.

His account under III.20 is nearly the same, except that here (as in other places) he makes it clear that this is no mere theoretical knowledge: he calls them now samyag-darśana-prāpta and a-prāpta. Samyag-darśana (Right Vision) is his strongest term for Knowledge-as-experience. He describes these kṣatriya Knowers (vidvāṃsāh) as engaged in going to Liberation (mokṣam gantum pravṛittāh) without abandoning action, thus fulfilling their past karmic involvement (prārabdha-karmatvāt).

The explanations under IV.14 and 15 are similar: the Self-knowers (ātma-jñā) or truth-knowers (tattva-vid) are seekers of Liberation (mumukṣu) but may continue in activity for the sake of the world.

Additional reasons why Knowers may continue in active involvement with the world are given here and there. Under III.21–25, Kṛṣṇa recommends vigorous action as an example to people at large.

Related to this may be 'to avoid the displeasure of the learned' (śiṣṭha-vigarhaṇāparijihīrṣā) under IV.20. This is probably a reference to Manu, who allows pursuit of Knowledge at any stage of life, but forbids pursuit of Liberation till the 'debts' to ancestors, etc. have been discharged through a householder's life.

There are blanket phrases like kutas nimitta and kutaścit nimitta '(from) some cause' in the commentary to IV.22: '... finding that for some reason it is impossible to abandon action ...'

Again, in VI.31 and XIII.23 there is the phrase about the Knower: 'however he may behave' (sarvathā vartamāno 'pi); and in V.7 'though doing, he is not tainted' (kurvann api na lipyate).

In these and other cases Śaṅkara cites prārabdha-karma, and/or lokasaṅgraha.

There are borderline cases. The instruction to fight 'as an instrument' is implemented at the end of the Gītā in the consciousness, according to Śaṅkara, 'There is nothing for me to do' (na mama kartavyam asti).

It is noteworthy that in his commentary, when enjoining renunciation of actions on a Knower, Śaṅkara frequently quotes V.13. In line-for-line translation it would be:

> Renouncing all actions by the mind, he sits happily in control,
> The embodied in the citadel of nine gates, neither at all acting nor causing to act.

He cites this (sometimes the second line) in his commentary to II.21, III.1, V.19, VI.l, XVIII.10, 48 (twice), and 66.

He explains that an appearance of action remains as a result of unspent karma. He could easily have quoted from the Gītā texts on outer renunciation as a reflection of inner renunciation, for instance XII.19: 'silent, content with anything, homeless....' But he chose this V.13 text, on renunciation by distinguishing mentally between action and non-action, and not necessarily entailing as corollary a physical renunciation. This is an indication of Śaṅkara's recognition that the Gītā is mainly a text for those who begin yoga when already heavily implicated in obligations in the world. They are not to be loaded with impracticable injunctions to renounce all physically.

www.ingramcontent.com/pod-product-compliance
Lightning Source LLC
Chambersburg PA
CBHW060308030426
42336CB00011B/969
* 9 7 8 1 9 1 1 4 6 7 1 5 1 *